100 Cases in Psychiatry

Second edition

100 Cases in Psychiatry

Second edition

Barry Wright MBBS FRCPsych MD
Professor of Child Mental Health University of York, UK

Subodh Dave MD FRCPsych
Associate Dean, Royal College of Psychiatrists, UK

Nisha Dogra BM DCH FRCPsych MA PhD
Professor of Psychiatry Education and Honorary Consultant in Child and Adolescent Psychiatry, University of Leicester, UK

100 Cases Series Editor:

Janice Rymer
Professor of Obstetrics & Gynaecology and Dean of Student Affairs, King's College London School of Medicine, London, UK

CRC Press
Taylor & Francis Group
Boca Raton London New York

CRC Press is an imprint of the Taylor & Francis Group, an **informa** business

CRC Press
Taylor & Francis Group
6000 Broken Sound Parkway NW, Suite 300
Boca Raton, FL 33487-2742

First issued in hardback 2018

ISBN 13: 978-1-138-37376-1 (hbk)
ISBN 13: 978-1-4987-4774-5 (pbk)

Library of Congress Cataloging-in-Publication Data

Names: Wright, Barry (John Barry Debenham), author. | Dave, Subodh, author. |
Dogra, Nisha, 1963- author.
Title: 100 cases in psychiatry / Barry Wright, Subodh Dave and Nisha Dogra.
Other titles: One hundred cases in psychiatry | Hundred cases in psychiatry |
100 cases
Description: Second edition. | Boca Raton, FL : CRC Press/Taylor & Francis
Group, [2017] | Series: 100 cases | Includes bibliographical references
and index.
Identifiers: LCCN 2017002751| ISBN 9781498747745 (pbk. : alk. paper) | ISBN
9781498747752 (e-book) | ISBN 9781315380483 (e-book)
Subjects: | MESH: Mental Disorders | Case Reports
Classification: LCC RC465 | NLM WM 40 | DDC 616.890076--dc23
LC record available at https://lccn.loc.gov/2017002751

Visit the Taylor & Francis Web site at
http://www.taylorandfrancis.com

and the CRC Press Web site at
http://www.crcpress.com

CONTENTS

PREFACE

Mental health problems are not confined to psychiatric services. It is now well established that significant mental health problems occur across all disciplines, in all settings and at all ages. Doctors need to be equipped to recognise these difficulties, treat them where appropriate and refer on as is necessary. All doctors need the knowledge and experience to sensitively enquire about such difficulties, to avoid the risk of problems going untreated.

This book does not provide an alternative to meeting real people and their families firsthand, which we would thoroughly encourage. This second edition provides clinical scenarios that allow readers to explore the limits of their knowledge and understanding, and inform their learning. These scenarios provide a vehicle where students and junior doctors can build their confidence in assessment and management. They are written in a way that encourages the reader to ask more questions, and seek the solutions to those questions. We hope that this book complements and adds an additional dimension to learning.

ACKNOWLEDGEMENTS

Thanks to the following people for their helpful contributions.

Additional case contributions:

Dr Mary Docherty, MBBS

Dr Simon Gibbon, MBBS, MRCPsych

Dr David Milnes, MBChB, MRCPsych, MMedSc

Dr Puru Pathy, MBBS, MRCPsych

Dr Mark Steels, BMedSc, MBBS, MRCPsych

Proofreading and additional contributions:

Dr Jeff Clarke, MBBS, FRCPsych

Dr Bhavna Chawda, MBBS, MRCPsych

Dr Ananta Dave, MBBS, MRCPsych

Dr Khalid Karim, BSc, MBBS, MRCPsych

CASE 1: HOW CAN YOU ASSESS MENTAL STATE?

History

A 42-year-old woman comes into hospital for a laparoscopic cholecystectomy. The admitting doctor has concerns about her mental state. There are concerns about whether she is healthy enough to cope with an operation and the recovery from it. The doctor takes a psychiatric history.

Question

In addition to the history what assessment will give more information about this woman's mental health, before a decision about whether to proceed with surgery or whether to ask a psychiatrist to see her?

ANSWER 1

The mental state examination is equivalent to the physical examination in medicine or surgery, but a different system is being examined. It takes place through observation and through probing questions designed to elicit psychopathology. It is structured and follows a procedure. It is put together with the history and investigations. The mental state examination contributes to the formulation, which is a summary of the mental health problems and their relation to other aspects of life. Formulation includes a diagnosis and may include a multi-axial diagnostic understanding (see Cases 24 and 79). Formulation uses information from the history and mental state examination to describe the three Ps: predisposing factors, precipitating factors and perpetuating factors. The mental state examination includes

Appearance: assess this woman's appearance. Look at hygiene, clothing, hair and make-up. Do the clothes suggest any subcultural groups? Are there any signs of neglect, perfectionism or grandiosity?

Behaviour: observe behaviour throughout. Look for evidence of rapport or empathy. Are movements slow or rapid? Is she agitated or is there psychomotor retardation? Each may be a possible signal for disorder. For example, the latter may be a sign of depression, hypothyroidism or parkinsonism. Are there invasions of personal space seen in autism spectrum disorders, mania, schizophrenia and personality disorder? Does the person sit still or move about? Is the person calm, or impulsive and distractible? Is the person monitoring or watchful of anything and if so what? A spider phobic may be looking out for spiders; a person with schizophrenia may be listening to unseen voices; a person with obsessive-compulsive disorder may be carrying out rituals in relation to the environment; a person with autism spectrum disorder may be examining environmental detail.

Speech: assess the volume, flow, content, pitch and prosody of speech. A person with mania may be loud, have flight of ideas, pressure of speech and use puns. A person with schizophrenia may be 'un-understandable' if he or she has formal thought disorder. There may be limited speech or short answers in depression, hypothyroidism or with negative symptoms of schizophrenia. A person with autism spectrum disorder may have little communication or may speak only on one subject at length with poor conversational reciprocity.

Mood: assess what this is like subjectively and objectively. How does the person describe his or her mood and is it congruent with what you see and experience in the room? This will include questions about enjoyment, worthlessness, hopelessness, suicidality and risk (see Case 33).

Thoughts: assess content and whether there is any formal thought disorder, or evidence of rumination or intrusive thoughts. Do thoughts race as in mania? Are they negative as in depression? Are they resisted as in obsessive-compulsive disorder? Are they interfered with as in the thought passivity of schizophrenia (see Cases 16 and 42)? Assess beliefs such as delusions (see Case 16) which can occur in psychosis, dementia and organic brain damage.

Perception: assess perceptual experiences by observation and questioning. Is the person responding to the visual hallucinations of delirium tremens or organic brain disorder, or the auditory hallucinations of schizophrenia, organic illness or psychotic depression? Are perceptions heightened as when abusing certain drugs or dulled as when abusing other drugs? Are there pseudohallucinations as in bereavement? Hallucinations (see Case 16) are important markers of mental illness.

Cognitive function should be carefully assessed (see Case 64) and will uncover organic disorders or the pseudodementia of depression. Do they have capacity (see Case 73)?

Finally assess *insight*. Who/what do they attribute their problems to? How do they see their problems and the need for treatment?

Key Points

- Mental state examination is the equivalent of an examination of a physical system, but is an examination of the mind.
- It is more than a history. It requires careful observation.

CASE 2: HE DOESN'T LISTEN TO ME

History

A 43-year-old pharmaceutical representative has been referred by his general practitioner (GP) as he is concerned that he may be suffering from attention deficit hyperactivity disorder (ADHD). His elder son, 11, was diagnosed with ADHD at the age of 8 – the same age when he recalls developing his own symptoms.

He has been reading up about ADHD and has completed an online screening tool. He recalls being a *hyperactive* child – he had difficulty playing or engaging in leisure activities quietly, often spoke excessively and out of turn, was constantly fidgeting and squirming when seated in the class, would make frequent excuses to leave the classroom or when at the cinema and was generally 'running about' everywhere as if 'wired to a motor'. He also recalls being quite *impulsive* and impatient, so much so that he had difficulty waiting in line for his turn and would blurt out responses out of turn. He remembers being disorganized and *inattentive* – he was easily distractible and had difficulty focusing or concentrating; he was constantly making silly errors in school work, losing things and had difficulty completing assignments on time.

His hyperactivity has calmed down over the years though he still finds it difficult to relax when doing nothing and can feel quite restless when inactive. He has changed several jobs and finds himself getting bored easily. He often comes up with 'brilliant ideas' in team meetings but has poor motivation in following them through. He starts many new projects but then fails to complete them. He finds it hard to carry out mundane tasks: he has never managed to claim his travel expenses and tends to become drowsy in lectures or more worryingly when driving long distances. His 360-degree feedback at work included positive comments about his inexhaustible energy and initiative but also referred to his failure to complete tasks and his tendency to talk over others or to become quite impatient and frustrated with colleagues.

At home, his wife complains that she has to mother him and that she is like his personal assistant – organizing things for him, finding things that he has misplaced and reminding him of his responsibilities. She feels particularly upset about the fact that he doesn't listen when she is speaking to him and she has to constantly repeat what she has said to him. He has been irritable at home and his wife is contemplating a separation. He enjoys adventure sports and 'online shopping binges' but has periods when he gets sullen and withdrawn. He does not misuse tobacco, alcohol or any other illicit substance.

Examination

Physical examination is unremarkable. On mental state examination, he appears worried and anxious to be given a diagnosis of ADHD. His mood is euthymic but he seems fidgety during the interview. There is no thought or perceptual disturbance.

Questions

- What is the differential diagnosis?
- What treatments should you offer?

ANSWER 2

The clinical picture is strongly suggestive of ADHD. He reports at least five symptoms of inattention (avoiding mundane tasks, having difficulty finishing projects, losing belongings, being easily distractible and failing to listen to others in conversation). He developed symptoms of inattention, hyperactivity and impulsivity before the age of 12 and his symptoms are pervasive (seen both in his home and work environments). They have led to significant disturbance in socio-occupational functioning (negative feedback from colleagues; threat of separation from his wife). The diagnosis can be confirmed by obtaining corroborative history from parents or teachers. Self-rating scales such as Conners, Adult ADHD Rating Scale can be helpful. It would be important to check GP records in childhood for ADHD assessment, Child and Adolescent Mental Health Services (CAMHS) involvement or other relevant information such as school problems, minor injuries etc. This man's symptoms cannot be better explained by another psychiatric or medical disorder or by substance misuse. Adult ADHD is the most appropriate diagnosis based on *Diagnostic and Statistical Manual of Mental Disorders, Fifth Edition* (*DSM-5*) criteria. Bear in mind the possibility of feigned or exaggerated symptoms (e.g. for drug misuse). Symptoms of hyperactivity and impulsivity may subside in adulthood and in this case symptoms of inattention are prominent.

ADHD continues into the teens in two-thirds of children and of these a further two-thirds will retain the disorder in adulthood. It is associated with significant co-morbidity in adults; the most common co-morbid diagnoses are anxiety disorders, depression or bipolar disorder which are the main differentials. Medical disorders such as thyrotoxicosis should also be ruled out. Substance (stimulants) misuse is of particular concern especially in vulnerable populations such as patients in prisons.

Methylphenidate is the first-line treatment in adult ADHD according to National Institute for Health and Care Excellence (NICE) guidelines. Treatment should be initiated with a low dose of 5 mg tds and the dose can be gradually increased over 4–6 weeks based on treatment response and side effects up to a maximum of 100 mg/d in doses divided three or four times a day. Modified release preparations should be given no more than twice a day and ideally once a day. Atomoxetine or dexamfetamine should be considered if adequate trial with methylphenidate does not produce a response. Medication treatment requires close monitoring for side effects – cardiac side effects with stimulants (methylphenidate and dexamfetamine) and behavioural effects such as irritability and suicidal thoughts with atomoxetine. Stimulants are controlled drugs and prescribers should therefore be familiar with controlled drug legislation in their jurisdictions. In practice, treatment is likely to be prescribed by specialists rather than by primary care practitioners.

Psychological treatments without medication should only be considered if drug treatments are not acceptable or not effective. However, the care plan should address psychological, behavioural, educational and occupational needs of the patient and in this case referral for marital counseling and a referral to individual or group cognitive behaviour therapy (CBT) to help improve organizational skills may be appropriate.

Key Points

- ADHD can persist into adulthood and can have significant impact on social and occupational functioning.
- Methylphenidate is the treatment of choice in adult ADHD.

CASE 3: 'STRESSED'

History

A 40-year-old schoolteacher attends his general practitioner surgery with his wife with complaints of feeling constantly fearful and stressed. These feelings have been present on most days over the past 3 years and are not limited to specific situations or discrete periods. He also experiences poor concentration, irritability, tremors, palpitations, dizziness and dry mouth. He has continued to work, but his symptoms are causing stress at work and at home. He denies any problems with his mood and reports that his energy levels are fine. He admits that he is experiencing problems with his sleep. He finds it difficult to fall asleep and states that he does not feel refreshed on waking up. He has been married for 15 years and lives with his wife and two sons aged 8 and 10. His parents live locally and he has no siblings. His father has been diagnosed with Alzheimer's dementia. He remembers his mother being anxious for much of his childhood. He has no previous medical or psychiatric history and is not taking any medication. He smokes 20 cigarettes per day and drinks alcohol socially. He has never used any illicit drugs. He tends to hide his symptoms and said that he was seeing his general practitioner because his wife wanted him to seek help.

Mental state examination

He makes fleeting eye contact. He is a neatly dressed man with no evidence of self-neglect. He appears to be restless and tense but settles down as the interview progresses. He answers all the questions appropriately and there is no abnormality in his speech. His mood is euthymic and he does not have any thoughts of self-harm. There is no evidence of delusions or hallucinations. He is able to recognize the impact of his symptoms on his social and occupational functioning and is keen to seek help.

Physical examination

His blood pressure is 140/90 mm Hg and his pulse is regular and 110 beats per minute. The rest of the physical examination does not reveal any abnormality.

Questions

- What is the differential diagnosis?
- How would you investigate and manage this patient in general practice?

ANSWER 3

This man is suffering with generalized anxiety disorder (GAD). His predominant symptom is a feeling of constant fear and insecurity. He also has symptoms of anxiety related to autonomic arousal including tremors, palpitations and a dry mouth. These symptoms have been present on most days for a period greater than 6 months. These symptoms are constant and not limited to specific situations like fear of being embarrassed in public (social phobia), fear of heights (specific phobia), discrete periods (panic attacks), or related to obsessions (obsessive-compulsive disorder [OCD]) or to recollections of intense trauma (posttraumatic stress disorder [PTSD]).

! Differential diagnoses

- *Depression*: Anxiety symptoms are common in depression and co-morbid depression is often seen with GAD. The type of symptom that appears first and is more severe is conventionally considered to be primary.
- *Panic disorder*: There is a discrete episode of intense fear with sudden onset and a subjective need to escape.
- *Other anxiety disorders*: They have the same core symptoms as in GAD but the symptoms occur in specific situations as in phobic anxiety disorder, OCD or PTSD.
- *Substance misuse*: Symptoms of alcohol or drug withdrawal may mimic those of anxiety.
- *Physical illness*: A host of medical conditions can mimic GAD – endocrine disorders such as hyperthyroidism or phaeochromocytoma; neurological disorders such as migraine; deficiency states such as anaemia or vitamin B_{12} deficiency; cardiac conditions such as arrhythmias and mitral valve prolapse; and metabolic conditions such as hypoglycaemia and porphyria.

A detailed history and mental state examination are needed to rule out the differential diagnoses listed above. Relevant blood tests like thyroid function tests, blood glucose and complete blood count are needed to rule out the physical differentials. Additional tests can be done in the context of other findings on history or examination.

Patients seen in early stages of GAD may respond to counselling offered in primary care. Those with moderate to severe symptoms need cognitive behaviour therapy (CBT), which is the first-line treatment. Chronic or severe cases may need referral to psychiatric services, as in the case of this patient. Anxiety management provided by a community mental health nurse is often effective and no other treatment is needed. Selective serotonin reuptake inhibitors (SSRIs) such as fluoxetine, paroxetine or citalopram can be useful but may cause paradoxical increase in agitation and reduce patients' concordance with treatment. Side effects should be monitored carefully. Benzodiazepines carry a risk of developing tolerance and dependence with continuous use and should only be used very rarely and then for no more than 3 weeks.

Key Points

- GAD is characterized by a constant feeling of fear and insecurity.
- CBT is the treatment of choice. Benzodiazepines should be avoided.

CASE 4: SICK NOTE

History

A 43-year-old medical representative attends the general practice surgery requesting a sick note. She is due to deliver a presentation next week to the national team, upon which hinges her hope of a promotion. She says that the thought of doing this presentation is making her feel very panicky. She has always had stage fright and even the thought of speaking in public makes her tremor worse. When asked to speak in public or when making presentations to doctors or nurses, she develops palpitations, sweating, dizziness and a feeling of butterflies in her stomach. She feels that she will make a fool of herself in public and therefore goes to great lengths to avoid such situations. When she has had to make presentations in the past to her local team, she has used a 'couple of drinks' to calm herself. She is single and is particularly nervous about dating. She feels that her problems have worsened over the past 3 years since she was promoted to hospital representative. Since then she has tended to fret about forthcoming presentations and her sleep has been quite poor. Over the last week she has been extremely agitated and has found it hard to concentrate on anything, so much so that she nearly had a serious road traffic accident. Fortunately, she escaped with a dent in her car. She reiterates her request for a sick note, as it would be 'impossible' for her to do the presentation. She would like to drive down to see her sister in Cornwall instead. There is no evidence of recurrent sick notes in her medical notes.

Mental state examination

She is a well-dressed woman wearing make-up. She establishes a good rapport and is cooperative. She appears very fidgety and restless. She is sweating profusely and keeps fanning herself with a magazine. Periodically, she gets tearful and her voice becomes tremulous. Her mood is clearly anxious and agitated. She does not have any formal thought disorder or indeed any other psychotic symptoms. She is a little irritable and gets upset when she feels that her request for a sick note is not being taken seriously. She has good insight into her symptoms. She acknowledges that she has not sought help 'all these years' but expresses her willingness to try any treatment that is likely to work.

Physical examination

Physical examination is unremarkable apart from tachycardia of 100/min.

Questions

- How will you deal with her request for a sick note?
- What advice do you give her in relation to her driving?

ANSWER 4

This lady is presenting with somatic and psychological symptoms of anxiety, which seem to occur in specific social situations where she fears she will embarrass or humiliate herself. So far, she has coped with these situations either by self-medicating with alcohol or by avoidance of the anxiety-provoking situation. The most likely diagnosis is either social phobia or panic disorder, although co-morbid depression needs to be ruled out, as do alcohol misuse or endocrine problems.

Presently, she is very anxious about a presentation at work and is requesting a sick note. Sick notes for physical illness are usually less problematic as objective evidence of illness is often available. Stigma about psychiatric illness, both from the patient and the doctor, can further create barriers to providing a sick note. The presence of drugs or alcohol in the clinical narrative, as is the case here, can make one take a judgemental view. Parsons' concept* of the *sick role* suggests that sick people get sympathy and are exempt from social obligations such as work or school. In return, however, there is the expectation that they will seek help and accept the offered treatment. This lady is likely to respond to cognitive behaviour therapy (CBT) but that may take weeks. Similarly, selective serotonin reuptake inhibitors (SSRIs) such as fluoxetine may be effective but are unlikely to help her next week. Benzodiazepines can relieve anxiety in the short term but carry the risk of dependence as well as cause drowsiness and sedation. This lady has a clinical diagnosis of an anxiety disorder and is willing to accept treatment. A sick note should help reduce the stress she is experiencing. It is important, however, to ensure that the sick note does not become an avoidance mechanism that tends to reinforce the underlying anxiety. The sick note should therefore be time limited and supported by efforts aimed at helping her back to work and engaging with treatment.

! Driver and Vehicle Licensing Agency

Anxiety or depressive disorders, unless severe, do not usually necessitate suspension of driving. Effects of medication for these conditions or symptoms that impair driving must however be judged on an individual basis. With psychotic disorders (e.g. schizophrenia or mania) the Driver and Vehicle Licensing Agency (DVLA) guidance requires suspension of driving during the acute illness and for 3 months after complete resolution of the acute episode. Return of the license requires that the patient is compliant with treatment, that treatment side effects do not impair driving, that the patient has regained insight, and that the patient has a favourable specialist report. Fitness to drive is also usually impaired in dementia.

This lady has significant problems with concentration and agitation, which are impairing her ability to drive. DVLA guidance requires her driving to cease pending medical enquiry with resumption after a 'period of stability', which needs to be judged clinically. She should be advised not to drive. If she refuses to heed this advice, General Medical Council (GMC) guidelines advise breaking confidentiality and informing DVLA.

Key Points

- Stigma about psychiatric illness may hamper return to work; sick leave relieves stress in the short term, but prognosis improves with return to work.
- The DVLA needs to be informed if the patient continues to drive despite being unfit to do so.

---

* Parsons T. 1975. The sick role and the role of the physician reconsidered. *The Millbank Memorial Fund Quarterly* 53, 257–278.

CASE 5: CHECKING

History

A 27-year-old man presents with a 6-month history of increasing repetitive routines. He is now unable to leave the house without undertaking lengthy repetitive checking of locks, taps and switches. He is taking longer and longer so that he is often late for work. He is worried about losing his job as other colleagues have been made redundant. He had a similar episode when he was 18 around the time of his 'A level' examinations but that settled within a few weeks which is why he has delayed seeking help. He wants to know what is wrong with him and what treatment options there are that do not require medication.

Mental state examination

His eye contact is good. He is anxious and gently rubs his hands together without looking at them. His mood is not low subjectively or objectively. His speech is normal. There are no delusions or hallucinations and nothing else of note.

Questions

- What is the most likely diagnosis?
- What are the treatment options?
- What are the Key Points about the therapy you would need to make sure the patient is aware of?

ANSWER 5

The most likely diagnosis is obsessive-compulsive disorder (OCD). OCD can take many forms, but, in general, persons experience repetitive, intrusive and unwelcome thoughts, images, impulses and doubts which they find hard to ignore. These thoughts form the obsessional part of 'obsessive-compulsive' and they usually (but not always) cause the person to perform repetitive compulsions, which are attempts to relieve the obsessions and neutralize the anxiety. Often there is a thought about completing an action that is accompanied by a fear that if they do not comply something dreadful will happen. They recognize that their fears and anxious behaviours are irrational but they do not stop themselves acting on them.

Medication is not recommended as a sole treatment method but is often used as an adjuvant treatment if the patient is willing. Research has shown selective serotonin reuptake inhibitors (SSRIs) are most effective for OCD, for example fluoxetine, fluvoxamine, paroxetine, and sertraline are the first line of treatment, but in the case of these being ineffective, clomipramine and others may be tried. Medication sometimes work by reducing the severity of the obsessive-compulsive symptoms or by 'taking the edge off' some of the anxiety precipitated by OCD. Cognitive behaviour therapy (CBT) is a tried and tested treatment. CBT helps patients change how they think ('cognitive') and what they do ('behaviour'). CBT focuses on the 'here and now' problems and difficulties. It does not seek to look at the past for causes for current behaviour and feelings (Figure 5.1).

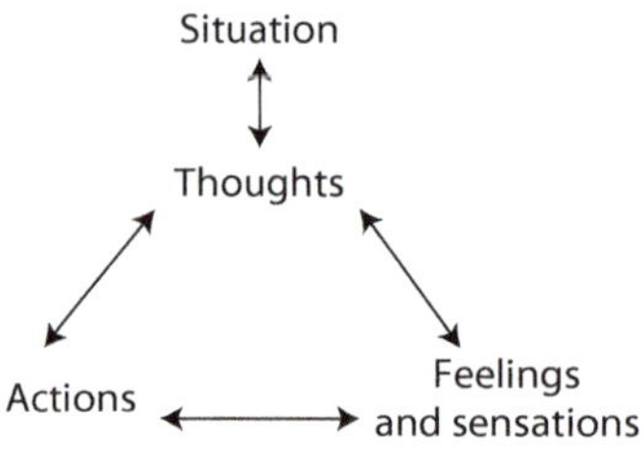

Figure 5.1 Simple CBT interactions.

In this case he will need to consider how the obsessive thoughts lead to certain other thoughts, sensations, feelings and actions. CBT recognizes how these aspects interact in reinforcing cycles. It can help change how this man responds to his thoughts and feelings leading to alternative outcomes and a reduction in distress.

CBT can be done individually or with a group of people. It can also be done from a self-help book or computer programme. CBT can be time consuming and needs motivation and commitment from the patient. Treatment usually involves 5–20 sessions weekly or fortnightly and sessions vary between 30 and 60 minutes. The problem is broken down into separate parts. It is usual to keep a diary to help identify individual patterns of thoughts, emotions, bodily feelings and actions. The relationship between these components is explored and techniques devised to help change unhelpful thoughts and behaviours. There is usually some 'homework' or 'experiments' between sessions, and this may include diaries. As an example, response prevention is practised where compulsions are not carried out with discussion of thoughts, feelings, actions and outcomes. Meetings are used to do cognitive work, carry out and plan experiments and review how the tasks were undertaken and how further success can be built. CBT can be difficult to implement if someone is acutely distressed as it does need a level of clear thinking. Depression is often a co-morbid problem.

Key Points

- CBT is the treatment of choice in OCD.
- CBT is a time-consuming therapy that requires work and commitment from the patient outside of the therapy sessions.
- SSRIs are the first-line medications used and can be very effective.

CASE 6: HAVING A HEART ATTACK

A 36-year-old schoolteacher is brought in by the paramedics to the emergency department. This is her fifth presentation in 4 weeks. She woke up from her sleep last week drenched in sweat and experiencing an intense constricting chest pain. She reported a racing heart, difficulty breathing and an overwhelming fear that she was about to die. She called 999 (emergency telephone number in the United Kingdom) who took her to the emergency department where all investigations were normal. She was discharged with a diagnosis of 'panic attack' but she had a similar attack 2 weeks later. On her third presentation she was referred to a psychiatrist. She had another episode last week, which was managed by the paramedics.

Today, however, she said that the chest pain was far more severe and she was also feeling dizzy, choking, with hyperventilation, numbness and tingling in her left arm, which convinced her she was having a heart attack. The paramedics tried to reassure her but she started screaming and flailing her legs and arms forcing them to take her to the emergency department once again.

She tells you that she thinks she is dying or going mad. She is terrified of having another attack and has insisted her husband take leave over the past week to be with her. She refuses to go out anywhere without him. She is upset about having called 999 but says the emergency doctors saved her life. She is avoiding her bedroom as four of the five attacks have happened there. She is avoiding lying down and instead spends the night in her armchair. Her husband is extremely concerned. He is particularly worried as her father has a history of myocardial infarction and her mother has had a stroke. She has tried cannabis a few times, the last time being 6 months ago. She smokes when she goes out for a drink with her friends – usually once a month. They live in their own home, have no children and have no financial worries.

Physical examination

She appears calmer but shaken. She is drenched in sweat and still tremulous. She has tachycardia and tachypnoea, but blood pressure (130/84 mm Hg) is normal. There is no other significant abnormality.

Investigations

Her electrocardiogram is normal. Random blood sugar, thyroid profile, serum calcium and urine drug screen are also normal.

Questions

- What is the diagnosis and what are the likely complications?
- How will you explain the diagnosis and possible treatment to her and her husband?

ANSWER 6

This lady is presenting with a *panic attack* which is a discrete period of intense fear or discomfort developing abruptly and peaking within 10 minutes. It is characterized by palpitations, sweating, trembling, shortness of breath, choking sensations, nausea, abdominal distress, dizziness, fear of loss of control or 'going crazy', fear of dying, tingling sensations, numbness and chills or hot flushes. Derealization (feelings of unreality) and depersonalization (feelings of detachment from self) may also be seen. She has recurrent attacks with persistent fear of having another attack (fear of fear) and worry about the implications of having the attack (fear of heart attack and death) suggesting a diagnosis of *panic disorder*. She is anxious about sleeping at night and is *avoiding* her bedroom and is engaging in the *safety seeking* behaviour of going to the emergency department or of keeping her husband next to her. This suggests a diagnosis of *panic disorder with agoraphobia*.

Medical conditions that need to be ruled out include hyperthyroidism, hyperparathyroidism (serum calcium), phaeochromocytoma (hypertension with headaches, tachycardia), hypoglycaemia and cardiac arrhythmias.

Phobic avoidance and agoraphobia are common complications in panic disorder and can lead to the patient becoming housebound. Alcohol, substance misuse and depression are other possible complications.

Reassuring her and her husband that there is no serious physical illness is important but so is acknowledging the reality of her distress and the worry of her husband. Cognitive behaviour therapy with her will explain the link between emotions (fear), cognitions (belief that sleep may induce an attack) and safety (sleeping in the armchair) and how this is crucial as an explanation of the vicious cycle. It creates a link between sense of apprehension and physiological changes such as increased heart rate (see Figure 6.1). These bodily changes are interpreted catastrophically with fear of something awful happening (*catastrophic misinterpretation*) leading to more anxiety which leads to further sympathetic response and somatic symptoms perpetuating the vicious cycle. This explanation provides the basis for cognitive behaviour therapy which is the recommended treatment for panic disorder with or without agoraphobia. Recognizing signs of a panic attack and understanding the stress response can abort a panic attack. Cognitive therapy can be explained using the hot cross bun model pictured in Figure 6.2.

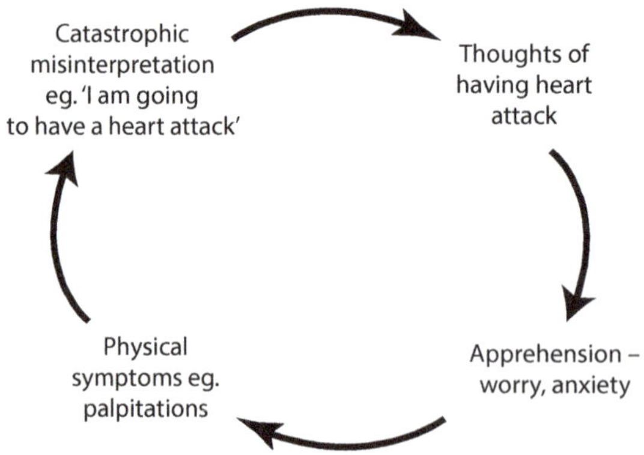

Figure 6.1 Panic attack.

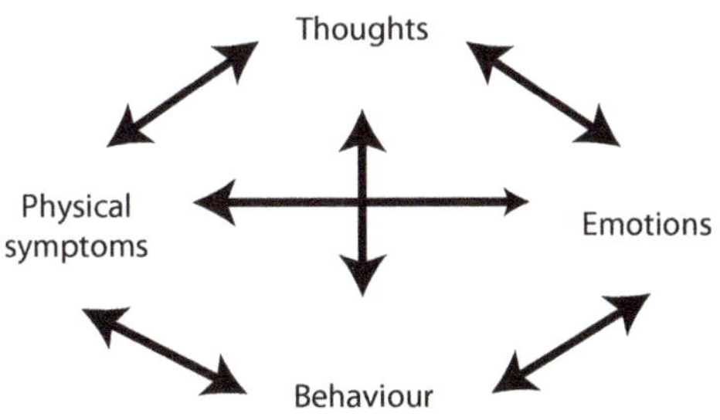

Figure 6.2 Cognitive therapy: the hot cross bun model.

Short-acting benzodiazepines such as alprazolam and lorazepam reduce the frequency and intensity of panic attacks but carry a high risk of dependence and are therefore not recommended. Tricyclic antidepressants such as imipramine and selective serotonin reuptake inhibitors (SSRIs) such as fluoxetine are effective though SSRIs may induce anxiety and agitation in the short term.

Key Points

- Repeated catastrophic presentation of anxiety symptoms in the absence of a medical cause suggests panic disorder.
- Reassure patients and significant others, explaining the link between physical and psychological symptoms.

CASE 7: GOING THROUGH A BAD PATCH

History

A 34-year-old bank manager attends the general practice surgery with her 8-year-old son, who is suffering from asthma. She appears tremulous and becomes tearful while talking about his problem. She says that she has been very worried about her son and has not been sleeping very well for the past 5–6 months. She has been eating reasonably well although she admits that she has felt more tired and demotivated than usual. She is still going to work but has found it hard to concentrate on her work as well as before. She worries that she might make a serious mistake at work. She says that she has managed to cope with the support of her husband, who has been 'a rock'. However, there have been days when she has found it difficult to get out of bed. She feels she is going through a bad patch and is hopeful that things will get better soon. She does not see a problem with her self-esteem and finds her work enjoyable but exhausting. She completely dismisses any idea of self-harm or suicide, saying she would never even think about it. She apologizes profusely for becoming emotional and asserts that she is normally very calm and composed but had been overcome by the stress of her son's illness. She requests a glass of water and takes a few deep breaths as her 'heart was beating fast'.

She lives with her husband in their own four-bedroom house. There is no family history of any major medical or psychiatric illness. In particular, she denies history of any mood episodes, either depression or hypomania. She drinks alcohol socially, never exceeding 10 units per week. She does not smoke or use any illicit drugs. She describes herself as a 'go-getter'. She is a keen runner and runs 12–16 miles a week.

Physical examination

She agrees to a brief physical examination. She has a tachycardia of 108 beats per minute, her pulse is regular and her blood pressure is 138/88 mm Hg. Her palms appear cold and sweaty but there is no other significant physical finding.

Mental state examination

She is pleasant, cooperative and establishes a good rapport. She is clutching her son protectively but maintains good eye-to-eye contact throughout the interview. Her speech is of normal rate and volume. Her mood is anxious and low. She does not have any psychotic symptoms. She has a good insight into her symptoms. She does not wish to take any medications but acknowledges that she needs to be 'strong' to be able to look after her son. She does not have any ideas of self-harm.

Questions

- What are the possible diagnoses?
- How should this woman be managed?

ANSWER 7

This woman is presenting with a mixture of anxiety and depressive symptoms occurring in the context of her son's illness. She is feeling very stressed and has coped well with her husband's support. Diagnostic possibilities include

- Mixed anxiety and depression. This is a common presentation in primary care characterized by a mix of anxiety and depressive symptoms without clear prominence of any one type and the presence of one or more physical symptoms (typically tremor, palpitations, lethargy etc.) present for more than 6 months.
- Adjustment disorder with depressed mood or with mixed anxiety and/or depression. This occurs in reaction to a stressful event or situation usually lasting less than 6 months with onset within 3 months of onset of a stressor. The symptoms are not caused by bereavement and the symptoms do not persist for more than an additional 6 months after cessation of the stressor.
- Depression. She does have the core symptoms (low/anxious mood, reduced energy) and some other symptoms (reduced concentration, poor sleep) lasting more than 2 weeks suggesting a mild depressive episode.
- Other disorders that need exclusion include generalized anxiety disorder or medical causes of anxiety/depression. Dysthymia (characterized by depressed mood over 2 years and two or more from a list of reduced or increased appetite, insomnia or hypersomnia, low energy, low self-esteem, poor concentration and feelings of hopelessness) can be excluded in this case due to the duration criteria. Bipolar disorder needs to be excluded by asking about hypomanic/manic episodes.

Detailed history and mental state examination will be needed to establish the diagnosis. Appropriate investigations to rule out any medical disorders will also be required. National Institute for Health and Care Excellence (NICE) guidelines suggest that when depressive and anxious symptoms coexist, the first priority should usually be to treat the depression. Psychological treatment for depression often reduces anxiety, and many antidepressants also have sedative/anxiolytic effects.

A stepped care model approach would be well suited to this situation. This woman has mild mood symptoms and as per the stepped care model, these are best treated initially in a primary care setting. 'Watchful waiting' (follow-up appointment within 2 weeks) with reassurance is sensible, as symptoms may resolve spontaneously. If symptoms persist on subsequent visits, brief psychological interventions may be provided by the practice counsellor or primary care mental health worker. Computerized cognitive behaviour therapy (CBT), healthy lifestyle advice about exercise and sleep hygiene are also helpful. Guided self-help using manuals or self-help books are other options available in primary care. If her symptoms worsen, treatment can be commenced taking into account her preference. She can be referred for primary care-based psychological treatments such as CBT (e.g. Integrated Access to Psychological Therapies [IAPT] in England). Alternatively, if she prefers (or if CBT has proven to be unsuccessful), antidepressant/anxiolytic medication such as selective serotonin reuptake inhibitors (SSRIs) can be effectively administered in primary care.

Treatment-resistant cases, psychotic symptoms, atypical symptoms or recurrent episodes should trigger a referral to specialist services. At any stage, if risk profiles change rapidly and risk assessment indicates a risk to self, to others or of self-neglect a referral can be made to the crisis team for consideration of inpatient treatment.

Key Points

- Establish the diagnosis and severity of mood disorder.
- Manage mild/moderate cases in primary care using a stepped care approach.

CASE 8: I'M PUTTING WEIGHT ON

History

A 19-year-old health care assistant attends the psychiatry outpatient clinic for her first follow-up since discharge. She had been admitted with the first episode of paranoid delusions, running commentary hallucinations and has been diagnosed with paranoid schizophrenia. She has been prescribed olanzapine 15 mg daily. Her psychotic symptoms have been effectively controlled with this medication. She is no longer experiencing any positive psychotic symptoms (see Case 15) and does not report any significant negative symptoms either (see Case 31).

However, she has gained nearly 6 kg in weight over the 3 months that she has been taking olanzapine. She is 1.5 m tall and her baseline weight was 52 kg (body mass index [BMI] increase from 23 to 25.7). She used to smoke 20 cigarettes a day but has recently switched to rolling her own and is using about 100 g of tobacco a week. She does not use any illicit substances. She drinks about two bottles of wine a week and acknowledges that she had no motivation to exercise following discharge. She is extremely concerned about this weight gain and is keen to discuss this during her appointment.

Mental state examination

She is dressed smartly. She is pleasant, articulate and expressive. She does not have any psychotic symptoms. Her mood is euthymic. She understands the implications of her diagnosis and is keen on adhering to the prescribed treatment.

Physical examination

Her blood pressure is 128/78 mm Hg. Her waist measurement is 33 inches. There is no remarkable finding on systemic examination. Her blood investigations were reported as being normal at the point of admission. Her latest investigations done the day before her clinic appointment are given below.

Investigations

	Levels	*Reference range*
Haemoglobin	13.4 g/dL	13.3–17.7 g/dL
Mean corpuscular volume (MCV)	85 fL	80–99 fL
White cell count	8.8×10^9/L	$3.9–11.0 \times 10^9$/L
Fasting plasma glucose	6.4 mmol/L	<6.1 mmol/L
Hb1Ac	44 mmol/mol (6.2%)	<42 mmol/mol (<6%)
Total cholesterol	5.6 mmol/L	<5 mmol/L
HDL cholesterol	0.8 mmol/L	>0.9 mmol/L (men) >1.0 mmol/L (women)
LDL cholesterol	3.7 mmol/L	<3 mmol/L
Fasting serum triglycerides	2.4 mmol/L	<2 mmol/L

Questions

- What is the explanation for the changes in her weight and in her investigations?
- How will you manage her?

ANSWER 8

This is a case of first-episode psychosis that is being managed with a second-generation antipsychotic medication, olanzapine. While these medications are less likely than the first-generation antipsychotics (see Case 41) to cause extrapyramidal side effects, they have been associated with significant metabolic side effects such as weight gain, impaired glucose tolerance and hyperlipidaemia. This woman exhibits dyslipidaemia (raised triglycerides and lowered HDL cholesterol), raised fasting glucose, and central obesity meeting four of the five criteria (barring raised blood pressure) needed for the diagnosis of metabolic syndrome. She has gained weight rapidly (>5 kg over 3 months) which along with her impaired glucose and lipid tests, places her in the red zone of the Lester Adaptation of the Positive Cardiometabolic Health Resource suggesting the need for immediate intervention.

People with schizophrenia have their life expectancy reduced by 15–20 years and cardiovascular disease (CVD) is the single largest cause of this premature mortality (more so than suicide) in this population. She has other risk factors that enhance this risk. She is a smoker (largest risk factor for CVD in people with mental illness), has become more sedentary since her discharge and is likely to need to remain on her antipsychotic medications. While 50% of patients commencing antipsychotic medications gain >7% of their body weight in the first 12 months (as she has), they are at continued risk of gaining further weight over the next 36 months.

The intervention in her case needs to target (1) smoking, (2) lifestyle, (3) weight and BMI, (4) blood pressure, (5) glucose levels and (6) blood lipids. There needs to be a proactive approach in collaboration with her, her primary care practitioner, the psychiatric care team and significant carers to maintain her physical health and well-being. She should be referred for smoking cessation counseling but given her increasing dependency may need specialist support to help her stop or reduce smoking. Nicotine replacement therapy and/or varenicline are known to be effective. She should be encouraged to contain her calorific intake and exercise regularly (moderate intensity, 30 min/d). Community-based weight and diet management programmes with periodic reviews (3-monthly in this case) of key parameters (weight, BMI, waist measurement, blood lipids, glucose, electrocardiogram) to encourage and maintain compliance with healthy nutrition and lifestyle changes will be useful.

In her case, she will need to be referred to a metabolic specialist given the diagnosis of metabolic syndrome. Hypertension, obesity and dyslipidaemia may require appropriate pharmacological treatment – NICE guidelines offer useful protocols. Given the rapid onset of metabolic syndrome in her case, her antipsychotic medication needs to be reviewed and consideration must be given to reducing the dose or to switching to an alternative medication. This decision must take into account the risk of relapse of psychosis and patient preference.

Key Points

- Metabolic syndrome reduces the life span of patients with schizophrenia.
- Medication review, lifestyle advice and appropriate specialist referral are needed.

CASE 9: UNRESPONSIVE IN THE EMERGENCY DEPARTMENT

History

A 30-year-old man is brought to the emergency department by his girlfriend in an unresponsive state. His girlfriend provides the history. She left him in his bedsit last night but found him lying unconscious this morning. She says that he has been an intravenous heroin addict for the past 5 years but is certain that he never shares needles and has had regular negative tests for HIV. In the past he has made several unsuccessful attempts to quit heroin, the last one being as recent as a week ago. There is no significant medical or psychiatric history. He is unemployed and lives on his own. His parents died when he was young, and he does not have any surviving relatives.

Examination

His pulse is 70 beats per minute regular, blood pressure 108/58 mm Hg. His respiratory rate is 10 breaths per minute. He is in a hypotonic hyporeflexic coma but there are no focal neurological signs. There is no verbal response though he groans in response to pain. His Glasgow Coma Scale (GCS) score is 4/15. His SpO_2 (percutaneous oxygen saturation) is 75%. He has pinpoint pupils. His arms and legs reveal multiple scarred needle puncture sites. His consciousness improves significantly (GCS of 15) following an intravenous bolus of 0.3 mg of naloxone.

Investigations

	Levels	*Reference range*
Haemoglobin	13.8 g/dL	11.7–15.7 g/dL
White cell count	9.8×10^9/L	$3.5–11.0 \times 10^9$/L
Sodium	138 mmol/L	135–145 mmol/L
Potassium	4.0 mmol/L	3.5–5 mmol/L
Urea	5.2 mmol/L	2.5–6.7 mmol/L
Creatinine	92 μmol/L	70–120 μmol/L
Bicarbonate	16 mmol/L	24–30 mmol/L
Glucose	4.0 mmol/L	4.0–6.0 mmol/L
Calcium	1.64 mmol/L	2.12–2.65 mmol/L
Arterial blood gases on air		
pH	7.29	7.38–7.44
PCO_2	7.4 kPa	4.7–6.0 kPa
PO_2	9.6 kPa	12.0–14.5 kPa

Note: Electrocardiogram: no abnormality detected; chest X-ray: normal.

Questions

- What is the immediate management?
- How will you manage him in the long term?

ANSWER 9

This man has the characteristic combination of impaired consciousness, bradypnoea and miosis indicative of opioid toxicity. Pinpoint pupils may be observed in pontine lesions or after local cholinergic drops, but history and examination suggest opioid overdose. Naloxone is a specific opiate antagonist with no agonist or euphoriant properties. On intravenous or subcutaneous administration it rapidly reverses the respiratory depression and sedation caused by heroin intoxication, confirming the diagnosis, as in this case. Immediate management involves securing the airway, stabilizing breathing and circulation (ABC) and providing supported ventilation and intravenous fluids. Naloxone is administered at a continuous 0.3 mg/h infusion aimed at keeping the GCS at 15 and a respiratory rate over 12 breaths per minute. He will need to be observed in an intensive care unit (ICU) with naloxone infusion until all opioids are cleared from the system. Investigations include blood and urine toxicology, full blood count for infections and arterial blood gases to monitor oxygenation. Further investigations include liver function tests, rapid plasma reagent (RPR), hepatitis viral testing, HIV testing in view of IV drug use and chest X-ray to rule out pulmonary fibrosis.

Detailed history and mental state examination are needed to assess whether the overdose was accidental or deliberate and to rule out psychiatric disorders such as depression. A sermon listing the ill-effects of substance misuse is likely to be ineffective and, in an acute setting, inappropriate. Motivational interviewing (MI) techniques have been shown to be more effective. This is where the patient, rather than the doctor, lists the costs and benefits of continued substance misuse. Key components of MI are as follows:

1. Using *empathy* to understand the patient's point of view and reasons for using opioids.
2. Allowing the patient opportunity to explore the *discrepancy* between positive core values (e.g. a desire to 'be good') and his or her unhealthy behaviours.
3. Tackling the inevitable *resistance* with empathy rather than confrontation.
4. Supporting *self-efficacy* and enhancing self-esteem.

Prochaska and DiClemente's stages of change* help identify the patient's readiness to engage in therapeutic change (see Figure 9.1).

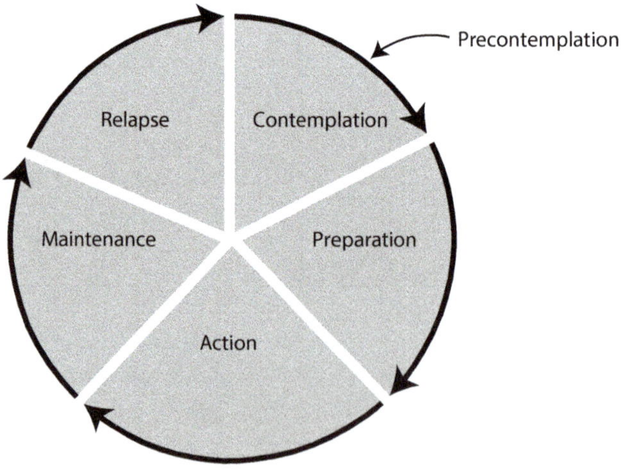

Figure 9.1 Stages of change.

* Prochaska JO, DiClemente CC. 1983. Stages and processes of self change of smoking: Toward an integrative model of change. *Journal of Consulting and Clinical Psychology* 51, 390–395.

The step-wise goals of treatment guide the patient through harm minimization strategies up to the complete cessation of the addictive behaviour. These include (1) reduce injecting; (2) reduce street drug use; (3) practice maintenance therapy (MT) with heroin substitutes methadone (long-acting μ receptor agonist) or buprenorphine (partial agonist); (4) reduce substitute prescribing; and (5) abstain. An ongoing psychosocial care package with cognitive or group therapy aimed at relapse prevention is vital. MT reduces illicit drug use, criminal activity, risk of seroconversion for HIV, hepatitis B and C and improves socialization. Methadone can be fatal in overdose and also has street value so medication is dispensed in liquid form (rather than tablets that can be reconstituted for injection).

Stages of change

Precontemplation: The patient does not acknowledge the problem and is often defensive about his or her substance misuse.

Contemplation: There is awareness of the consequences of substance misuse while weighing up of the pros and cons of quitting. There is no decision made to change.

Preparation/determination: A commitment is made to change, involving research and preparation for the consequences. Skipping this step and jumping to 'action' often leads to 'relapse'.

Action: Active efforts to change. It is boosted by external help and support.

Maintenance: Success in this stage involves avoiding relapse. This entails constant adaptation and acquisition of new skills to deal with changes in the environment.

Relapse: This is common and so it is useful to encourage a return to contemplation and re-entry into the cycle.

Key Points

- Opioid intoxication needs urgent treatment with naloxone, the opioid antagonist.
- Empathizing is more effective than sermonizing.
- MT reduces illicit drug use but must be supported with a full package of care.

CASE 10: FEELING EMPTY

History

A 34-year-old call-centre manager attends her general practitioner (GP) surgery with her boyfriend. She complains of tiredness and a lack of enthusiasm for life. These complaints started a year ago but have worsened over the past 2 months. She has been forced to take time off work as she was constantly arguing with the senior manager and found it difficult to remain calm and composed at work. She has also been irritable with her boyfriend, and gets upset easily if he tries to 'motivate' her. She knows that he is well meaning, but still finds it very irritating and yet feels guilty for responding to him in this way. She has lost all interest in sex or going out socializing. Despite being offered a great deal of support by her boyfriend, she constantly worries that he will leave her. Over the past 6 weeks when she has been at home, she has spent most of her time in bed. She admits shamefacedly that there are days when she does not wash or even brush her teeth. She vacantly watches the television, not able to take in anything. She feels 'empty' most of the time and finds it upsetting that she cannot even react to her boyfriend's efforts at reaching out to her. She watches TV until late finding it difficult to sleep. In the morning, she feels exhausted and tends to lie in bed until late. She has had thoughts of dying, but resists acting on these as she does not want to punish her boyfriend or her mother, who lives by herself.

She is an only child. She lives with her boyfriend in his flat. She is close to her mother and visits her weekly. Her father died following a stroke last year. She is healthy and has no medical problems. She does not drink or use drugs. She remembers being admitted to a psychiatric unit on a section at the age of 19 as she had become 'very high'. She remembers taking lithium for a while, but now has been off it for years. The only other psychiatric episode she can recall was on a holiday to Greece when she became quite elated and was convinced that she was Venus, the goddess of love. She went to the local market, topless, was arrested and admitted to a local psychiatric hospital. She was treated as an inpatient for 2 weeks and was discharged with some medication. She has only hazy memories of the episode, but remembers not taking the medication on her return to the United Kingdom.

Questions

- What is the likely diagnosis?
- How will you manage this patient in the short and longer term?

ANSWER 10

This woman is presenting with a moderate to severe depressive episode with a past history of two episodes of mood disorder, which appear to have been manic episodes (delusions of grandeur, elated mood and disinhibition requiring admission to an inpatient unit). The most likely diagnosis is bipolar disorder, with a current depressive episode.

To manage the current depressive element she should be referred to the mental health team for an urgent assessment. Antidepressants (on their own) may lead to a switch to mania, and should therefore be avoided. This is particularly so in cases of rapid cycling illness (more than four mood episodes per year) or in case of a recent manic episode. Psychotherapies such as cognitive behaviour therapy (CBT) or interpersonal therapy (IPT) may be helpful. Quetiapine on its own or fluoxetine combined with olanzapine are evidence-based treatments indicated to treat moderate to severe bipolar depression. Olanzapine or lamotrigine on their own are also useful and if the patient is already on lithium or sodium valproate, optimizing the dose within the therapeutic range may be helpful.

It is prudent to consider longer-term management. She has had more than two acute mood episodes, and therefore it is very likely that she will have further episodes of either depression or mania. Prophylactic treatment is strongly indicated in this case as it reduces the frequency and intensity of mood episodes. Lithium is the first-line treatment but if it is poorly tolerated or not suitable, then sodium valproate or olanzapine are recommended for prophylaxis; she is of childbearing age and therefore sodium valproate in particular and lithium are best avoided and should be prescribed only by specialists. Prophylaxis should be continued for at least 2 years after an episode, but may need to be as long as 5 years if risk factors such as severe psychotic episode, frequent relapses, co-morbid substance misuse, ongoing stress or poor psychosocial support are present. A key ingredient for a positive prognosis is patient engagement and self-management with self-monitoring of mood, early recognition of signs of relapse and prompt treatment. She and her boyfriend need to be actively involved with the psychiatrist and multi-agency team (community psychiatric nurse/occupational therapist) in developing a needs-based care plan including a crisis plan as they will be in the best position to identify early signs of relapse. Helping her with potential triggers such as shift work, improving sleep hygiene and providing extra support at times of stress is important. Advance directives can be useful in treatment planning for future episodes, as insight is often impaired in manic episodes and in severe depression. A shared protocol of care between primary care and secondary care is needed, and she should be offered regular physical health checks to monitor the physical health effects of her prophylactic medication. Weight, blood glucose, lipids, blood pressure, smoking and alcohol status should be monitored regularly. Her boyfriend may benefit from a carer's assessment and referral to a support group.

Key Points

- Identification of bipolar depression is crucial as management is different from that in unipolar depression.
- Psychoeducation with identification of a relapse signature is crucial in ameliorating future episodes.
- Relapse prevention planning should be part of care for any major mental illness.
- Monitoring physical health is vital especially when prophylactic medication is prescribed.

CASE 11: I DON'T WANT PILLS, I WANT SOMEONE TO TALK TO

History

A 36-year-old stockbroker attends the general practitioner (GP) surgery requesting help with her mood. She has been feeling very stressed and has been finding it difficult to cope with work. She is used to working in a high-pressure environment but now feels burnt out and is worried that she may lose her job. She broke up with her boyfriend of 6 years 9 months ago and has been single since then. She has little interest in dating but has been having casual sexual relationships, which only make her feel worse about herself. She feels guilty for having neglected her boyfriend on account of her work, but also feels angry with him for having abandoned her. She cries to sleep every day and tends to wake up early. She has little interest in anything, but forces herself to go to work though it leaves her feeling exhausted so that she spends the weekend in bed. She hates herself physically, thinking she is too fat. She says she hates her personality as she believes she is too dependent and clingy.

She feels desperate about the future fearing that her biological clock is ticking away. She feels very guilty about a medical termination of pregnancy that she had with her boyfriend and feels that she can never forgive herself for having the abortion. There is no significant medical history. She has never formally sought help for any mental health problems, but feels that she has lacked in confidence for years.

She is close to her mother and visits her daily. She says that her father walked away from the family when she was 13 years old. She has refused to meet him though her two brothers have made peace with him. She feels that since then she became a gloomy pessimistic person. She thinks that her friends and colleagues perceive her as a critical, humourless person. She had a brief course of cognitive behaviour therapy (CBT) in the past and although she engaged, she found it unsatisfying because she felt it focused more on the present, when she was wanting to talk about her father and other past issues, which she felt were unresolved.

She lives on her own in her apartment. She drinks two bottles of wine over the weekend, but does not see this as a problem. She does not smoke or abuse any illicit drugs.

Mental state examination

She is dressed smartly wearing subtle makeup. She establishes a good rapport and is very deferential. She speaks articulately but starts sobbing when talking of her abortion. She looks visibly upset when talking about her boyfriend. Her anger is evident when talking about her father. She clearly describes ideas of hopelessness, guilt and worthlessness. Her mood is low, but she does not have any ideas of self-harm. She has very good insight and she understands the need to deal with her symptoms and the personality issues underlying them. She is motivated to seek and to comply with any interventions. However, she would prefer not to take medication and requests a talking therapy.

Questions

- What psychological therapy would you prescribe her?
- How would you explain the role of psychodynamic therapy in her case?

ANSWER 11

This woman is presenting with low mood, tiredness, ideas of hopelessness, guilt and worthlessness with sleep disturbance of more than 2 years' duration. This is superimposed on long-standing traits of pessimism and low self-esteem. She may be suffering from a moderate depressive episode although underlying dysthymia characterized by at least 2 years of low-grade depressive mood also needs to be considered. Depressive episode superimposed on dysthymia is called *double depression*. National Institute for Health and Care Excellence (NICE) guidance recommends CBT for depression. However, the guidelines do state that 'psychodynamic psychotherapy may be considered for the treatment of the complex co-morbidities that may be present along with depression'.

This woman has experienced a series of losses in her life: her father, her unborn baby, her boyfriend and now possibly her job. She is motivated to change and is psychologically minded, i.e. is demonstrating an awareness of the psychological issues underlying her problems. This makes her a good candidate for psychodynamic therapy. The key feature of psychodynamic therapy is to understand current symptoms in the light of past experiences. The hypothesis is that unresolved conflicts arising from past relationships (e.g. in her relationship with her father in this case) create anxiety. In an effort to prevent this anxiety, the unconscious mind devises strategies that ward off anxiety-provoking thoughts and emotions that are too difficult to be dealt with in the conscious mind. These strategies are known as defence mechanisms. In moderation such strategies can be effective (and can be very useful in the short term) but when used excessively, they can contribute to psychopathology. For example, the defence mechanism of denial can prevent a person moving on developmentally or can mask other compensatory problems such as alcohol misuse. Psychodynamic work involves making links between past traumatic experience, defence mechanisms and current symptoms. This process is helped by encouraging the patient to engage in free association, which involves the patient talking freely without any censorship. Identifying obstacles to free association helps identify defence mechanisms such as denial or suppression which have led to the exclusion of painful material from the conscious mind. Analysis is also helped by an understanding of transference, whereby the patient transfers, to the therapist, emotions and beliefs about significant people in her own life. The therapist remains passive and neutral, facilitating the patient to talk freely.

Psychodynamic therapy may be provided in an individual or group setting. Psychoanalysis is an intensive therapy focused on developing detailed insight into the unconscious processes underlying the symptoms leading to a modification of personality. Sessions are conducted daily or several times a week and can last in excess of 2 years. Brief psychodynamic therapy, on the other hand, is time limited, often no more than 20 sessions, and focuses on a specific problem, for example, on the theme of loss in this case.

Key Points

- Psychodynamic therapy is useful in the case of mood and anxiety disorders with co-morbid complexities such as personality problems.
- It involves understanding current symptoms in the light of past experiences.
- Defence mechanisms are unconscious strategies evoked to prevent anxiety; however, in the long term they may worsen psychiatric symptoms.

CASE 12: NEVER FELT BETTER

History

A 33-year-old phlebotomist presents to the emergency department with his girlfriend to get a repeat prescription of his antidepressant citalopram. He seems very restless, pacing up and down the waiting room. He is mumbling to himself and intermittently starts singing rather loudly. He is wearing bright clothes and lots of jewellery. The girlfriend states that he used up 4 weeks' worth of medication in 2 weeks. When the staff nurse approaches him to calm him, he starts shouting and swearing loudly and becomes quite intimidating and threatening.

He was first diagnosed with depression 5 years ago and responded well to citalopram 20 mg once a day, which was discontinued after a year. Six months ago he became depressed once again and was again prescribed citalopram 20 mg a day. He has been seen every 4 weeks at the general practitioner (GP) surgery since then and has been quite well. On his last visit 2 weeks ago he complained of poor sleep and was prescribed temazepam 10 mg nocte (at night). He has been taking double the dose of his antidepressant of his own accord.

For the past 2 weeks he has had broken sleep, but despite that he feels full of energy. He has been off work for the past week as he was working on a breakthrough invention 'that would revolutionize phlebotomy'. His girlfriend is concerned about him as he has been very talkative and has been spending excessively and buying her vastly expensive gifts.

There is no adverse medical history and no other psychiatric history apart from the depressive episodes. He lives with his girlfriend. His parents live locally, he is an only child and there is no family history of mental illness. He smokes 15–20 cigarettes a day and engages in social drinking using no more than 10 units a week. He uses cannabis 'now and then' and has used cocaine in the past.

Examination

His eye contact is not good when you are talking but is intense when he is addressing you. He is talking quite rapidly and claims to be the 'Crown Prince of England'. He answers in rhyming ditties and breaks down in sobs holding his girlfriend's hand. He gets angry that he is not addressed as 'His Majesty' and becomes quite agitated. There are no hallucinations. He has little insight, but is willing to take antidepressant medication. He does not have any ideas of self-harm. Physical examination is unremarkable.

Questions

- What is the differential diagnosis?
- How would you investigate and manage this patient in the emergency department?

ANSWER 12

This man is presenting with a manic episode. He displays irritable mood, grandiosity, reduced need for sleep, psychomotor agitation and excessive spending reflecting poor judgement for 2 weeks. His symptoms have caused him to miss work and he meets the criteria for a current manic episode. He has had two episodes of depression and therefore meets the criteria for bipolar disorder currently in mania. He has been using extra doses of antidepressant medication and this may have precipitated the manic episode.

! Differential diagnosis of manic episode

- *Hypomania.*
- *Drug-induced manic episode*: Apart from antidepressants, other medications such as steroids and stimulants may cause manic episodes. Illicit drugs such as cocaine, amphetamines and hallucinogen intoxication can cause manic episodes and alcohol withdrawal may also mimic a manic episode.
- *Organic mood disorder*: Manic episodes can occur secondary to medical conditions such as stroke, hyperthyroidism or Cushing disorder and more rarely space-occupying lesions such as meningioma or gliomas.
- *Schizophrenia*: This is characterized by mood-incongruent delusions, hallucinations and prominent psychotic symptoms as opposed to mood symptoms.
- *Schizoaffective disorder*: Mood symptoms and schizophrenia symptoms are equally prominent.
- *Acute confusional state*: The agitation and affective lability seen in acute confusional states may mimic a manic episode.

Investigations

- Obtain collateral history from previous records and GP notes and detailed history from girlfriend.
- Conduct a detailed mental state examination to rule out formal thought disorder, mood-incongruent delusions and hallucinations suggestive of schizophrenia. A cognitive abnormality would be suggestive of delirium (acute confusional state).
- Conduct a urine drug screen to rule out intoxication with drugs such as amphetamines that may cause a manic episode.
- Perform blood tests such as whole blood count to rule out infection as a cause for delirium, urea and electrolytes to exclude an electrolyte imbalance causing delirium and thyroid function tests to rule out hyperthyroidism.

He is demanding more antidepressants which probably precipitated his manic episode. Discontinue his antidepressants and explain to him that they are likely to make him worse not better. He is acutely agitated and grandiose and is displaying impaired judgement. Agitation may be treated with a short-acting benzodiazepine such as lorazepam 1–2 mg orally or intramuscularly (IM) up to a maximum of 4 mg in 24 hours. If agitation is severe olanzapine 5–10 mg orally or for even faster onset of action olanzapine 10 mg IM up to a maximum of 20 mg/24 hours can be used. To avoid the risk of respiratory depression parenteral benzodiazepine should not be given until at least 1 hour after IM olanzapine administration. This man is exhibiting symptoms of a manic episode, and he should be referred for an assessment by the specialist psychiatric team. This would be either the mental health liaison team, crisis team or the on-call psychiatrist. An acute manic episode is typically treated with lithium or an atypical antipsychotic such as olanzapine, risperidone or quetiapine. Management should involve the least restrictive options appropriate to the situation, and thus the crisis resolution home treatment team should perform a risk assessment to consider whether home treatment is suitable. If not, informal admission needs to be offered. If this is refused, involuntary admission under the appropriate section of the Mental Health Act (MHA) needs to be considered (Section 2 in England and Wales).

Key Points

- Antidepressants may precipitate a manic episode and should be stopped.
- A risk assessment would determine whether home treatment or informal admission to hospital is appropriate. The Involuntary detention using appropriate legislation may be appropriate when risk to self or others is present.

CASE 13: ACHES AND PAINS AND LOSS OF INTEREST

History

A 52-year-old medical secretary visits her general practitioner (GP) surgery with a 3-month history of back pain, generalized body ache and tiredness. She feels absolutely exhausted and has found it difficult to go to work. She feels so tired and uninterested that she has stopped her usual weekend visits to her daughter and grandchildren. The pain is located in the lower back and is described as a constricting non-radiating pain, which seems to be better when she is lying down. However, she has difficulty falling asleep and often wakes up early in the morning. At times she continues to lie in bed until early afternoon. The pain in her back and her body ache do seem to get better as the day goes along. Her husband has been concerned about her as she is usually a 'go-getter'. She feels preoccupied with her pain, does not enjoy the taste of food and has lost weight, which is one 'silver lining to the cloud'. At work, she has again been slow and not as 'efficient' as she normally is. She has taken paracetamol and ibuprofen without much benefit.

Physical examination

There is no localized tenderness or inflammation and systemic examination is normal.

Mental state examination

Her eye contact is within normal limits but her face is expressionless. She appears slow, tired, takes a long time to answer questions and her voice is soft. She reports feeling 'empty' and lethargic with little interest in work or previously pleasurable activities. She reports feeling guilty at not wanting to see her grandchildren. She has difficulty concentrating but does not report a problem with libido. She does not have any thought disorder. She does not report any periods of elevated mood or any symptoms of anxiety.

Investigations

	Levels	*Reference range*
Haemoglobin	13.2 g/dL	11.7–15.7 g/dL
Mean corpuscular volume (MCV)	87 fL	80–99 fL
Erythrocyte sedimentation rate (ESR)	9 mm/h	<10 mm/h
White blood cell count	7.2×10^9/L	$3.5–11.0 \times 10^9$/L
Thyroid-stimulating hormone	3.5 mU/L	0.3–6.0 mU/L
Free thyroxine	13.9 pmol/L	9.0–22.0 pmol/L

Note: Rheumatoid factor: negative; anti-DNA antibodies: negative.

Questions

- What is the likely diagnosis?
- What factors will improve the likelihood of making the correct diagnosis?

ANSWER 13

This woman is presenting with multiple somatic symptoms of 3 months' duration. While ruling out an appropriate physical pathology is important (arthritis, for example, in this case), it is equally important to rule out depression, which is a treatable reversible disorder.

! Diagnostic criteria for depression

- Core symptoms: low mood, reduced energy and anhedonia (lack of interest and enjoyment)
- Cognitive symptoms: reduced concentration, ideas of helplessness/hopelessness/worthlessness, ideas of self-harm/suicide, reduced self-esteem
- Somatic symptoms: reduced sleep (especially early morning awakening), reduced appetite or weight loss, reduced libido
- At least two of the core symptoms along with three other symptoms for at least a 2-week period suggest a diagnosis of depression

Somatic syndrome is a specific subtype of depression characterized by at least four of the following: (1) loss of interest or pleasure, (2) lack of emotional reactivity to normally pleasurable surroundings and events, (3) waking in the morning 2 hours or more before the usual time, (4) depression worse in the morning (diurnal variation in mood), (5) psychomotor retardation or agitation, (6) loss of appetite and/or weight (often defined as 5% or more of body weight in the past month), or (7) marked loss of libido.

Less than a third of cases of depression are diagnosed in primary care. Knowledge of depressive symptoms does not seem to be an issue. It may be that patients do not discuss symptoms (feelings of hopelessness), feel it is embarrassing or stigmatizing (fear of labels, medication or admission) or present with symptoms that redirect attention elsewhere (e.g. somatic presentation, alcohol or substance use, anxiety disorders or complicated grief). Somatic presentation seems to be a key factor with diagnosis rates three times less when there is no obvious psychological factor in the presentation, as in the case of this woman. A simple rule of thumb is to ask screening questions for depression when there are three or more somatic symptoms irrespective of their cause. Somatic presentations have been reported to be more common in certain ethnic minorities; however, somatic presentations are common both in primary care and in secondary care where in specialties such as neurology, rheumatology or cardiology up to 40% of patients may present with medically unexplained symptoms.

Diagnosis improves with good communication skills in the doctor: better eye contact, open-ended questions, re-contextualizing physical symptoms to psychological causes using questions such as 'are you experiencing any stress?' or 'do you think these symptoms may be due to stress?'. Allowing enough time is important, and this patient should be offered a longer appointment to explore her symptoms in depth.

Key Points

- Depression may often present with somatic symptoms in primary care.
- Screen for core symptoms of depression when there are three or more somatic symptoms present.

CASE 14: CONSTANTLY TEARFUL

History

A 26-year-old woman complains of being constantly tearful for no clear reason that she can identify. She feels that given she has just had her first baby she should be feeling on top of the world. She reports that her recent pregnancy and birth were straightforward and she had been looking forward to the arrival of the baby. She is married and has good family support. The baby is fine although feeding has been difficult to establish.

Mental state examination

The woman looks red-faced and tired. She makes good eye contact. She is tearful. She says that her thoughts are tending to focus on worry about the future and the baby, but that she can also laugh and enjoy herself when she sees people she is close to. She can smile at interview. She has no hallucinations or delusions and has no thoughts of harm to herself or the baby. She believes her symptoms are present because she is exhausted.

Questions

- What further information do you need to make a diagnosis?
- What is the likely diagnosis?
- How would you manage this case?

ANSWER 14

The main considerations are whether this is 'baby blues' or whether something more serious is going on such as puerperal depression or puerperal psychosis. Establish how long ago the woman gave birth and consider the symptoms of baby blues (below). Given the symptoms and the absent history of depression it is most likely that this woman has the 'baby blues'. These are often linked to hormonal changes 3 or 4 days after delivery as pregnancy hormones drop and milk production begins. Sleep deprivation and exhaustion inevitably play their part. There are large emotional, social, family and practical adjustments to be made when a very dependent baby arrives within a family, and this may be very daunting. It is always important to exclude the more serious postnatal depression especially if more time has elapsed since the birth of the baby (e.g. 3 or 4 weeks). You will find that a proportion of women with postnatal depression will have also been depressed at some point in the last year when a good history is taken.

Baby blues affect 60%–80% of women usually appearing after the third day post-partum and resolving within a week.

Symptoms of baby blues

- Low mood
- Emotional distress and lability
- Tearfulness
- Over-sensitivity
- Anxiety
- Irritability
- Fatigue
- Difficulty sleeping
- Worry about minor problems
- Poor concentration
- Some mothers have pains for which there is no obvious medical cause
- Being unwell generally with no apparent cause and symptoms

There may also be anxiety about being a mother and looking after the baby. These feelings are within the range of normal feelings for women who have recently given birth. They last only a few days but can still be quite frightening especially if they take the woman by surprise.

No treatment is necessary other than reassurance, support from family and friends, rest, and time. A mother who has the blues should get as much rest as possible. Affected mothers may be over-sensitive about what is said to them by relatives and medical staff, so reassurance and tact and empathy from the staff can be very beneficial at this time. The tearfulness and anxiety will usually settle without any intervention. It is important however that the situation is monitored as, if the symptoms do not settle or are accompanied by suicidal thoughts, then the diagnosis may need to be reviewed. It is also important to watch for any difficulties in looking after the baby's needs. If the symptoms are severe or persist beyond 2 or 3 weeks after the birth, more active treatment may be warranted and the patient should be reassessed.

Key Points

- Baby blues is very common but is short lived.
- Reassurance and support are usually all that is required.
- Reassessment is useful to monitor progress.
- The baby's welfare should be monitored.

CASE 15: VOICES COMMENT ON EVERYTHING I DO

History

A 24-year-old man presents to casualty having got into a fight as he thought he was being watched and felt threatened. He appears to have fractured his thumb but is reluctant to let you examine him or order an X-ray. He looks suspicious and wary. When asked about his concerns he says that over the last few months he has been carefully monitored by government agencies. He has been hearing a voice out loud giving a running commentary on his thoughts and these are being broadcast to the government. Any machine enables the government to get inside his head and the voice is telling him it would be unwise to face the X-ray machine. The voice is not one that he recognizes, and it is sometimes derogatory, telling him he is stupid for giving his thoughts away for free. Initially the voice came and went but over the last few weeks it is present almost constantly and he cannot always sleep because even when he sleeps the voice comments on what he is thinking. He is exhausted.

The man is absolutely convinced that the government is after him but he cannot explain why. There is no previous history and he denies any substance use. Until a few weeks ago he had been working as a kitchen assistant but was sacked for leaving jobs unfinished. There is no family history of any psychiatric illness.

Mental state examination

The man looks unkempt. He is wary and looks quite frightened and agitated. His eye contact is fleeting and he constantly looks around him in a perplexed manner.

His speech is rambling and he does not express himself coherently. He occasionally uses words that you have not heard before and repeats them as though they have some significance. He does not come across as depressed. He has delusions of persecution. He has auditory hallucinations that provide a running commentary on every aspect of his behaviour. He has thought broadcast and thought withdrawal. He is orientated in person, but unclear about the time. He seems aware that he is in hospital but not quite sure why.

Questions

- What is the likely differential diagnosis in this case?
- What is the significance of the running commentary?
- What other symptoms may be commonly associated with this type of auditory hallucination?

ANSWER 15

The differential diagnoses are schizophrenia, schizoaffective disorder, drug-related psychosis and organic medical conditions. To make a diagnosis of schizophrenia, the symptoms and signs should be present for at least 1 month (as per *International Classification of Diseases, Tenth Revision* [*ICD-10*] criteria) and impact upon social and occupational or educational functioning. The following are usually present: delusions, hallucinations, formal thought disorder, 'negative' symptoms and abnormal behaviour.

A delusion is a firmly held idea that a person has despite clear and obvious evidence that it is untrue. Common delusions in schizophrenia include:

- Delusions of control: Belief that one's thoughts or actions are being controlled by outside, alien forces (passivity). Common delusions of control include thought broadcasting where private thoughts are being broadcast or transmitted to others, thought insertion (thoughts being planted in their heads) or thought withdrawal (thoughts being taken from their heads). Thought passivity is the terminology used to describe control of one's thoughts.
- Delusional perception: A real perception triggering a sudden delusional belief.
- Delusions of persecution: Belief that others are wanting to do the individual harm. These persecutory delusions often involve bizarre ideas and plots.
- Delusions of reference: A neutral environmental event is believed to have a special and personal meaning. For example, a person with schizophrenia might believe an innocuous phrase on TV is intended to send a message meant specifically for him or her.
- Delusions of grandeur: Belief that one is a famous or important figure or the belief that one has unusual powers.
- Somatic delusions are false beliefs about your body; for example, that a terrible physical illness exists or that something foreign is inside or passing through the body.

Hallucinations can be experienced in any of the sensory modalities and include:

- Auditory hallucinations (hearing voices in external space that other people cannot hear). Certain types of auditory hallucination are diagnostic of schizophrenia. These include hearing voices providing a running commentary on the person's behaviour or thoughts, two or more voices conversing with each other in the third person about the person, or if the individual hears his or her thoughts being echoed back.
- Somatic hallucinations (these suggest schizophrenia or an organic cause).
- Visual hallucinations (seeing things that are not there or that other people cannot see).
- Tactile, olfactory or gustatory hallucinations.

Formal thought disorder is a persistent underlying disturbance of conscious thought that is usually seen through spoken and written communication. This involves fragmented thinking experienced by the listener as being 'un-understandable' or the train of thought or associations between statements as disconnected. They may respond to queries with an unrelated answer, start sentences with one topic and end somewhere different, speak incoherently or say illogical things. There may be ongoing disjointed or rambling monologues in which a person seems to be talking to himself or herself or imagined people or voices. People with schizophrenia tend to have trouble concentrating. Some use neologisms, which are made-up words or phrases that only have meaning to the patient, or they exhibit perseveration, which involves the repetition of words and statements. Catatonic behaviour is sometimes present.

Negative symptoms reflect the reduction or absence of mental function and include reduced motivation, reduced use of speech and affective flattening.

Key Points

- Schneider first rank symptoms described in 1939 remain the cornerstone of the diagnosis of schizophrenia. They include:
    - Thought insertion, thought withdrawal and thought broadcasting
    - Running commentary, third-person auditory hallucinations and thought echo
    - Delusional perception, passivity phenomena, delusions of control and somatic hallucinations

CASE 16: I ONLY SMOKED A BIT OF CANNABIS AND TOOK A COUPLE OF Es

History

A 21-year-old man presents in an extremely frightened state. He is absolutely convinced that he has been followed and his life is at risk. When walking through town he was sure people were watching him, talking about him and planning how to kill him. He can trust no one including his friends. He has come to the hospital rather than go to the police because he believes the police are behind the conspiracy. He believes they have installed surveillance cameras in his flat and have been watching him. He feels others are jealous of his talents and success. He is convinced he has special powers and that is how he found out about the plots against him. He has had to start carrying a knife so he can protect himself from all his enemies.

The man has had no previous contact with psychiatric services and he has no medical history of note. All was well until the last few days. His sister recalls that about 6 weeks ago her brother and a few friends went to a music festival. She is aware that his friends have smoked cannabis and taken Ecstasy (E), but she thinks it is unlikely that her brother joined them. He does not smoke and has no prescribed medications.

The man is about to begin his final year at university. He has been studying physics and philosophy at university. He and his girlfriend finished their relationship just before the music festival. It was a reasonably amicable breakup, but had been a 3-year intense relationship. His interests include music and computer games. He has a good group of friends although over the last few days he has been avoiding them as he feels threatened by them.

Mental state examination

He is clearly frightened and suspicious, constantly looking around and trying to check what is going on. He makes intense eye contact when not looking elsewhere. He struggles to focus on the interview. His speech is rapid and his thoughts are not coherent. He jumps around from topic to topic. His mood is labile in that at times he seems to settle down but then quickly becomes alert and appears to be overactive. He has delusions of persecution and rather grandiose ideas about his own skills. He has auditory hallucinations, which tell him that he should kill if he needs to. He thinks the cameras in his house are being used to monitor his thoughts but he does not quite have thought withdrawal. He does not have any self-harm ideation. He is orientated in person in that he knows who he is, but he is not orientated in time or place. His short-term memory is poor and his long-term recall is variable as he is easily distracted.

Questions

- What is the differential diagnosis?
- How would you manage this man?

ANSWER 16

The differential diagnosis includes organic psychosis (given his age and recent circumstances drug-induced psychosis would be a high possibility), schizophrenia and bipolar disorder. Brief reactive psychosis may also be worth considering. In a reactive psychosis, psychotic symptoms may arise suddenly in response to a major stress, such as a death in the family or other important change of circumstances. Symptoms can be severe, but the person makes a quick recovery in only a few days.

With the short time frame it is likely that he has drug-induced psychosis. The acute management involves managing his risk. There is a moderate to high risk of him harming someone given his persecutory delusions. The fact that he thinks he is being watched and that his thoughts may be monitored means careful ongoing review is required to monitor his mental state. Given his delusions and the level of risk, hospitalization would be likely and medication may be necessary.

Using (or withdrawing from) drugs and alcohol can cause psychotic symptoms. Sometimes these symptoms will rapidly disappear when the drug is out of the system and the acute biochemical changes wear off. Psychotic symptoms usually occur during or shortly after (within 4 weeks) use of the substance. For some individuals, a predisposition to psychotic illness is triggered by the use of substances, particularly those that make more dopamine available at receptor sites such as amphetamines. However a range of other drugs may cause psychosis including alcohol, cannabis, LSD, cocaine, MDMA (Ecstasy) and withdrawal from benzodiazepines. It is important to realize that the trends in illegal substances are ever changing. Recently the use of 'legal highs' has been increasing. Legal highs are substances that have similar effects to illegal drugs like cocaine or cannabis. They are sometimes called club drugs or new psychoactive substances (NPS).

Although substance misuse is common, severe adverse reactions are much less common. Those at risk of developing problems should abstain altogether.

Key Points

- Drug-induced psychosis is usually brief but those who develop problems are at risk of developing the same symptoms if use continues.
- Some people with a vulnerability to schizophrenia may precipitate psychotic symptoms with substance use.

CASE 17: UNUSUAL PERSECUTORY BELIEFS

History

A 23-year-old electrical goods salesman attends his general practitioner (GP) surgery with his mother. He is very articulate but reluctant to talk, insisting that only the police can really help him. He explains that over the past 6 months his boss and his colleagues have conspired against him. Initially this was to dismiss him from his job but over the past few weeks they have conspired to kill him. He feels that they have been monitoring his activities and have even gone to the extent of bugging his flat and tapping his mobile phone. He is absolutely convinced of this and shows you some marks on the phone as evidence of it having been tampered with.

He insists, politely, that he will not allow a physical examination as this may present an opportunity to implant a microchip. In fact he is very worried that an old dental filling may be a transmitting device. He is preoccupied with these thoughts and is unable to distract himself. At work he feels constantly bombarded by his colleagues' nasty comments about him. He can hear them clearly even across the showroom. On one occasion he clearly heard derogatory voices from his manager's office on the other side of the building. He also knows that colleagues talk about him because of the way the price labels are arranged. His work has been affected. His boss has given him a performance warning and he sees this as further evidence of his boss's antipathy towards him. He feels that 'direct action' is now needed but he refuses to discuss this. He has contacted the police who have spoken to his colleagues. His mother indicates that the police say his colleagues admitted talking about him because his behaviour has been strange, but according to the police the charges of conspiracy are baseless and they have asked him to seek psychiatric help. His mother feels that his concerns are 'over the top' but does not feel that her son is 'psychotic'. She feels that he is under a lot of stress following a break-up with his girlfriend 6 months ago and pressure at work. His mother requests medication for him. He flatly refuses, but says that he will consider it if you 'endorse' his letter to the local Member of Parliament and the Prime Minister about the refusal of the local police to help him.

Questions

- How do you establish the diagnosis?
- How do you deal with his request?
- What do you tell the mother?

ANSWER 17

This man has a fixed belief that his colleagues are trying to kill him. Establishing that this idea is delusional involves proving that the belief is *false* or even if true held on false grounds (e.g. believing that colleagues are talking about him based on the arrangement of price labels). The belief is fixed and firmly held despite provision of evidence to the contrary and this is out of cultural norms. Gently challenging these ideas by providing evidence that is contradictory is vital in establishing the delusional nature of the belief. Providing alternative explanations, such as 'could the marks on the phone be accidental damage?', is an important part of history taking. So is further elucidation – 'I find it difficult to understand how a dental filling could act as a transmitter'. He has firm *conviction* in the delusional idea. Assessment of other dimensions such as *preoccupation, interference with work* and *acting out* reveal that he is preoccupied with these ideas and that this is affecting his work and that he is planning to act in response to his delusional ideas by 'direct action'. He is also hearing the voice of his colleagues across the showroom. Hallucinations have the quality of a true perception and occur in the absence of a real stimulus. It will be important to discover whether these are true hallucinations by verifying information about the showroom, the nature and content of the voices, and other examples that may be more clear-cut, such as hearing voices from a distant room while in the toilet. He has been experiencing culturally inappropriate and implausible delusions and apparent persistent auditory hallucinations for more than a month and therefore meets the diagnosis for schizophrenia.

His request involves colluding with his delusional ideas which may secure short-term gains, but in the long term it will betray his trust and damage therapeutic engagement. Empathizing with the true distress he is experiencing on account of his symptoms and offering to help him deal with his distress (even if there is disagreement about what is causing that distress) is likely to secure a better therapeutic rapport. However, he has mentioned 'direct action' and this will require a detailed risk assessment exploring both ideas of self-harm and of violence. If this direct action is proposed against his colleagues, the police should be informed even if it involves breach of confidentiality. In any case, an urgent referral to the local psychiatry team is indicated.

His mother is very worried for him and is probably concerned about the label of schizophrenia or psychotic illness. Providing education about the illness, providing leaflets, signposting to a patients'/carers' group or to a website such as www.rcpsych.ac.uk or www.rethink.org are likely to reduce expressed emotion (excessive hostility, criticism or over-involvement) in the mother. Expressed emotion is a known negative prognostic factor and risk factor for relapse.

Key Points

- Assessing delusions involves gentle challenging to establish firm conviction in the belief and assessing other dimensions such as acting out.
- Collusion with delusional ideas damages therapeutic engagement.
- Psychoeducation and engagement with carers is important to reduce expressed emotion.

CASE 18: ABDOMINAL PAIN IN GENERAL PRACTICE

History

A 26-year-old woman presents to her general practitioner (GP) with a complaint of abdominal pain. She has recently registered with this practice and is not known to this GP. She says that she has been experiencing discomfort in the epigastric region for the past 2 months and also complains of being bloated and being 'full of gas'. A year ago she had been referred to the specialist by her previous GP. She was investigated and an ultrasound examination of the abdomen revealed gallstones. She then underwent an uncomplicated laparoscopic cholecystectomy but has continued to experience the same pain. She says that the pain is present all the time and is not related to any particular foods. She complains of fatigue and breathlessness on minimal effort. She has been suffering from chronic back pain over the past 6 years. She had been seen by an orthopaedic specialist and underwent a magnetic resonance imaging (MRI) scan of the spine but no abnormality was detected. She attends regular physiotherapy sessions and has been using codeine phosphate 60 mg (up to four times a day) over the last 5 years. She has also presented on several occasions with bilateral knee pains and again investigations and specialist advice argued that there was no serious illness with a recommendation of normal exercise and good nutrition.

She is a single mother of two children aged 6 and 3 years. She lives in a two-bedroomed council flat, is unemployed and receives benefits. She has previously worked in a supermarket, a factory and a pub but did not hold any of the jobs for more than 6 months. Her relationships with the previous two partners (the fathers of the children) were volatile. Both partners had alcohol problems and were abusive towards her. She does not have any contact with her family and did not want to speak about them.

Examination of previous notes reveals that she has been a frequent attendee at her general practice. She has been investigated for urinary tract infections on several occasions but no evidence of infection has been found. She was referred to a gynaecologist at age of 18 with complaints of dysmenorrhoea, menorrhagia and was investigated for an ovarian cyst, and was given reassurance.

There is no previous psychiatric history. She smokes 20 cigarettes per day and drinks 10 units of alcohol per week. She has never used illicit drugs.

Mental state examination

She makes intense eye contact. She is dressed in bright clothes, talks about her symptoms animatedly and describes them in great detail. She is preoccupied with her various symptoms. She states that she feels low in her mood and admits that she finds it difficult to cope with her children. She has no thoughts of self-harm or suicide. She believes that the doctors have not been able to diagnose her problems and that she has been suffering due to their incompetence. She wants to be referred to a specialist for her abdominal pain.

Physical examination

There is no guarding or rigidity but she winces visibly on palpation of the abdomen. No other abnormality is detected.

Questions

- What is the differential diagnosis?
- How would you manage this patient?

ANSWER 18

This woman has symptoms suggestive of somatization disorder. She has multiple, recurrent and frequently changing physical symptoms that have been present for more than 2 years. She has undergone various investigations which have not been able to account for her numerous physical problems. She is preoccupied with her symptoms and has had multiple consultations with various health professionals. She has gastrointestinal symptoms (abdominal pain), cardiovascular symptoms (dyspnoea), genitourinary symptoms (investigations for urinary tract infection) and symptoms of pain. In patients suffering from this disorder there is often a refusal to accept reassurance that there is no medical reason for symptoms. Differential diagnoses to be considered include the following:

- Medical illnesses: Illnesses that may explain the patient's symptoms should always be ruled out before a diagnosis of somatization disorder is made.
- Depressive disorders: Patients with depressive disorder may experience somatic symptoms. This may particularly be a problem in people who have an inability to express emotions (alexithymia).
- Anxiety disorders: Symptoms of anxiety related to autonomic arousal can be mistaken for somatization. The autonomic nervous system itself can generate a range of real physical symptoms.
- Hypochondriacal disorder: In hypochondriasis there is a preoccupation with the fear of having a serious physical disease and often the patient refers to a particular illness by name.
- Intentional production of physical or psychological symptoms for assuming a sick role (factitious disorder/Munchausen syndrome) or for external purposes due to economic or legal reasons (malingering).

Detailed examination of previous medical notes to check the frequency of contact with health professionals and results of previous investigations help clarify the diagnosis. Relevant investigations may be needed to rule out physical illnesses that might explain the current symptoms. Patients should be dealt with in a sensitive manner without apportioning blame. It is important to reassure her that somatization does not imply that she is faking these symptoms. Some clinicians explain it as a close connection between mind and body, where stress in one domain can be experienced readily as real symptoms in another. A multidisciplinary approach would be required with emphasis on good communication between various professionals. Further follow-up should be with a single identified professional and it is important to discourage unscheduled appointments. The goal should be to build a rapport with the patient so that she is able to gain more insight into her symptoms and focus on any emotional triggers. The patient should always be informed before making a referral to a psychiatrist. Co-morbid depressive disorder may be treated with antidepressant medication and cognitive behaviour therapy may help with depression, anxiety or somatization.

Key Points

- Multiple somatic symptoms may indicate depression, anxiety or rarely somatization disorder.
- Rule out medical illness, malingering and factitious disorder (Munchausen syndrome).
- Avoid over-investigation and ensure all specialist reports are conveyed to all involved in treatment.

CASE 19: THERE IS SOMETHING WRONG WITH HIM

A 10-year-old boy presents with anxiety and refusal to leave the house unless both of his parents are with him. He is reported to have 'panic attacks' during which he hyperventilates as he struggles to breathe, feels dizzy and shaky. These can last up to 10 minutes or so and only seem to resolve when his parents reassure him that they will both stay with him until he is better. Although he is reluctant to go to school, he does attend as long as he is accompanied by both parents and is promised that they will be picking him up. When he is in school he is settled and there are no obvious features of anxiety. Staff note that he fits in well with peers and does not cause them any concern although he is academically a little behind. His parents are keen for their son to be offered individual therapy to help with his anxiety. Both parents have long-standing anxiety problems of their own but feel that they deal with these away from their son and he is unaware of their anxieties. They both feel that their son's anxiety is a significant factor in the stress that they are experiencing and they have begun wondering if they can continue with their marriage.

Questions

- What do you think the main problem here might be?
- How might you manage this situation?

ANSWER 19

Although the boy seems to be presenting with anxiety it should be evident that there are various family factors at play. Individual therapy of any sort is unlikely to be a helpful option in this case as even if the boy is anxious, the factors that maintain his anxiety will remain unaddressed. In a case such as this it is especially useful to apply the framework for considering predisposing, precipitating and perpetuating factors and then decide where treatment can be most effectively targeted.

Factor	Possible intervention	Comment
The genetic predisposition to developing anxiety.	Treatment targeted to specific genetic markers not available currently.	Awareness is helpful as this may allow an individual or family to plan to put coping strategies in place.
The features of anxiety that appear to be present.	These symptoms may cause alarm and evoke parental responses that perpetuate the presentation.	Can be unhelpful to get into debate about whether these symptoms are real or not as that rarely helps move the situation forward. It may be helpful to think of these as an expression of his distress.
Parental responses to initial anxiety may lead to specific behaviours.	Parent psychoeducation about anxiety and parental maintenance of clear expectations and boundaries through parenting programme: helping the parents change their ways of providing support – avoid giving reassurances or making blanket promises that perpetuate the problems.	It is important not to be critical of the initial strategies the parents may have used but to understand that they might have been the only strategies that were available at the time. The strategies the parents have used may have been initially helpful but their continued use has made them unhelpful as they have unintentionally maintained the problems.
Parental anxiety – may be predisposing in terms of genetic factors, but may also be precipitating and perpetuating.	Ensure that parental anxiety is being effectively managed through cognitive behaviour therapy, self-help programmes and psychoeducation.	Although the parents are insistent that their anxiety is kept from their son, most children are fairly aware when all is not well with the family. They will often imagine the situation is worse than it may be because they can only guess at what they are not being told.
Parental relationship difficulties may be precipitating and perpetuating.	Ensure the parents are aware of the impact of their relationship on their child.	Children pick up on parental tensions and in this case it may be that the boy is unconsciously becoming the glue in their relationship, e.g. by requiring both of his parents' presence to ensure that they do not separate.

Lack of clear communication in the family may serve as a precipitating and perpetuating factor.	Family work or family therapy.	Different members of the family may feel that in not raising issues they are helping the family but what may be happening is that there is much miscommunication and misunderstanding.
Being behind academically – this may be predisposing, precipitating and perpetuating.	This may mean that the boy has some learning difficulties or disability. Identify it and ensure the appropriate supports are in place.	The reason this factor may be predisposing is that if he is unable to understand information he may become anxious. Not understanding or misunderstanding familial issues may precipitate or perpetuate any features of anxiety.
Lack of any anxiety in school.	This is important as it indicates that individual therapy may be of limited benefit, but also that he can cope with his worries.	This highlights the need to look at the wider picture. The lack of anxiety in the school context supports the rationale for addressing the family issues as a priority.

Key Points

- A child's presentation to mental health services may reflect wider systemic issues that need addressing to help resolve or improve the situation.
- In assessing for child mental health presentations and their management, particular attention may need to be paid to the parental understanding and management of the child.
- It may be more challenging to gain parental agreement that the management of this case needs for work to be undertaken with them rather than with their son alone.

CASE 20: A DRINK A DAY TO KEEP MY PROBLEMS AT BAY

History

A 54-year-old man presents with abdominal pain for several days. The pain is a constant dull ache which is central and radiates to the right. He has had some associated vomiting but the vomit is usually bile as he has not been eating well. He has on a few occasions vomited some blood (haematemesis) but says that this was after particularly heavy consumption of alcohol. He is not aware how many units he drinks in a week but reluctantly admits he drinks every day. His breakfast often consists of a drink as he feels very shaky otherwise. Once he has had a drink he feels better able to manage the day ahead. He lives alone in a bedsit and eats poorly.

He says he was sacked for taking time off work for physical complaints. He has been separated from his wife for 6 months and no longer has regular contact with his children who he says have turned against him. The marriage had been difficult for some years because he was unable to hold down a regular job. He held a middle manager's post until he turned 50. Since then he has had a series of short-term junior posts. He believes that this is a result of changes in local government and not related to his drinking.

Physical examination

He has a ruddy complexion, several spider naevi on his face and red palms. He has a body mass index of 32. He is slightly tender in the right hypochondrium and lumbar regions and in the epigastric region of his abdomen.

Mental state examination

He smells of alcohol. He is reasonably well dressed. He looks unwell and is clearly uncomfortable. He has good eye contact. His speech is normal. He admits he has felt low as his life has deteriorated over the last few months but says he is not 'depressed'. He can still enjoy himself and is reactive at interview. He does not have any self-harm ideation. He has little hope for the future. There is no evidence of psychosis.

He is orientated in time, place and person. His short-term memory is poor but there are no long-term memory problems.

Investigations

	Levels	*Reference range*
Haemoglobin	12.4 g/dL	13.3–17.7 g/dL
Mean corpuscular volume (MCV)	109 fL	80–99 fL
White cell count	8.8×10^9/L	$3.9–11.0 \times 10^9$/L
Platelets	280×10^9/L	$150–440 \times 10^9$/L
Sodium	139 mmol/L	135–145 mmol/L
Potassium	3.5 mmol/L	3.5–5.0 mmol/L
Urea	2.3 mmol/L	2.5–6.7 mmol/L
Creatinine	75 μmol/L	70–120 μmol/L

Questions

- What might his liver function tests (LFTs) show?
- What are questions associated with the CAGE questionnaire?
- What are the features of alcohol dependence?
- What are the physical complications of alcohol problems?

ANSWER 20

His LFTs are likely to show the following:

- Elevation of alanine aminotransferase (ALT) also known as alanine transaminase.
- Elevation of aspartate aminotransferase (AST) also known as aspartate transaminase (two- to fourfold).
- ALT usually greater than AST (ratio of greater than 2 suggests alcoholic liver disease).
- A switch to AST greater than ALT may indicate cirrhosis.
- Likely to be elevations of gamma-glutamyl transpeptidase (GGT), alkaline phosphatase and ferritin.

LFTs in this man's case were as follows:

Investigations

	Levels	*Reference range*
Alkaline phosphatase	351 IU/L	30–300 IU/L
ALT	276 IU/L	5–35 IU/L
GGT	865 IU/L	11–51 IU/L
Bilirubin	24 μmol/L	3–17 μmol/L

The CAGE questionnaire

This asks the following key questions:

1. Have you ever felt you should *cut* down on your drinking?
2. Have people *annoyed* you by criticizing your drinking?
3. Have you ever felt bad or *guilty* about your drinking?
4. Have you ever had a drink first thing in the morning to steady your nerves or get rid of a hangover (*eye-opener*)?

The threshold for the CAGE suggesting potential problems is two out of four. It is clear in this case that this man has a significant problem. The following signs and symptoms strongly suggest *alcohol dependence syndrome*:

1. Strong desire to take alcohol with a narrowed repertoire of drinking.
2. Dominance of drinking over other responsibilities.
3. Tolerance to alcohol – that is, needing more and more alcohol to produce the same effects.
4. Physiological withdrawal state if alcohol is reduced or ceased.
5. Use of alcohol to prevent withdrawal.
6. Preoccupation with alcohol use and compulsion to drink.
7. Return to drinking even after periods of abstinence.
8. Persistence of alcohol use despite the harmful effects (may be physical, social or emotional).

There is often co-morbidity with other mental illnesses such as depression, social anxiety, anxiety, obsessive-compulsive disorder, other substance misuse and personality disorders.

The physical complications of alcohol misuse include liver disease such as fatty liver, alcoholic hepatitis or alcoholic cirrhosis. High blood pressure and other cardiac problems can occur especially if drinking is compounded by poor diet, low exercise and obesity. There is increased likelihood of cancer of the liver, stomach, colon, rectum, lung, pancreas, larynx and oesophagus. Pancreatitis, epileptic seizures and sexual dysfunction are also common. Abrupt abstinence in someone with alcohol dependence syndrome can lead to delirium tremens, which includes shaking, sweating, diarrhoea and seizures as well as hallucinations and an acute confusional state (see Case 26). This requires urgent medical attention as it can be life threatening.

Other physical signs in acute intoxication are slurred speech, dizziness, clumsiness, unsteadiness, blackouts, collapse and somnolence. Weight loss can occur with poor nutrition, or in end-stage disease. Peptic ulceration and pancreatitis can lead to abdominal pain. The skin can often give tell-tale signs including redness in the face or cheeks, rhinophyma, palmar erythema, hand 'liver flap' and numbness or tingling of the fingers. Malnutrition and pseudo-Cushing can also create distinctive changes.

It is common for social problems and family dysfunction to go hand in hand with alcohol dependence. This is clearly the case with this man. Given the complexity of this case and the seriousness of the presentation the safest way to manage him is likely to be through admission to enable both physical and mental health problems to be addressed.

Key Points

- Alcohol misuse has a range of physical, social and psychiatric complications.
- Listen carefully to how the CAGE questions are answered as many may be less than forthcoming.
- A significant number of acute medical admissions are directly or indirectly related to alcohol (including in the elderly).

CASE 21: PARACETAMOL OVERDOSE

History

A 24-year-old woman presents having taken an impulsive overdose of 30 paracetamol tablets. Earlier in the evening she had been drinking and ended up in an argument with her boyfriend. She returned home and thought about the evening. She felt very angry and unhappy and impulsively took the overdose. She is sure she did not take anything else. There is no suicide note and about half an hour after taking the overdose she called a friend who called an ambulance. She regrets the overdose and up until the argument with her boyfriend had not had any problems or issues that worried her. As a teenager she had a spell when she used to cut herself but this has not happened for at least 8 years. She has not taken any previous overdoses. She is rather embarrassed and upset.

Mental state examination

Her eye contact is normal. She looks well. Her speech is normal. She has no thought disorder. Her mood is stable and there is no current deliberate self-harm ideation. She does not express any feelings of hopelessness. She can enjoy herself and she has plans for the future. She has no evidence of any delusions or hallucinations. She has good insight into what has happened.

Questions

- What investigations, if any, would you do?
- How would you manage her?

ANSWER 21

The key questions are as follows:

- Is the patient presenting after a single or staggered overdose?
- What is the time of the ingestion?
- What are the blood tests showing?

An overdose of paracetamol (especially if greater than 7.5 g which is usually 15 tablets) that presents within 1 hour is treated using charcoal, which reduces gastrointestinal absorption. Early presentation of a paracetamol overdose is easier to manage than late presentation. If presentation is between 1 and 4 hours a blood test is required after 4 hours of ingestion to assess the levels of paracetamol. If there is any doubt about the drugs taken, it is always safest to err on the side of caution. Emergency departments have charts showing the relationships between blood levels and lengths of time since ingestion, and thresholds for further treatment. Access to TOXBASE, the primary clinical toxicology database of the National Poisons Information Service, is available online in all NHS hospitals and can be consulted for all up-to-date protocols in managing cases of overdose and poisoning.

Patients at increased risk of liver damage from lower blood levels of paracetamol include the following:

- Regular alcohol intake above recommended levels (14 units for women and 21 for men)
- Regular use of enzyme-inducing drugs (e.g. carbamazepine, phenytoin)
- Conditions including glutathione depletion (such as HIV, cystic fibrosis, eating disorders)

Hepatocyte damage can occur from metabolites of paracetamol breakdown including *N*-acetyl-p-benzoquinone imine, leading to liver failure. If the blood test after 4 hours indicates the need for treatment or there is uncertainty about the time of ingestion or the amount taken, the treatment is intravenous *N*-acetylcysteine. This replenishes glutathione, important in conjugating the damaging metabolites. Oral methionine can also be used for the same purpose.

In this case, she will require a blood test and may need treatment with *N*-acetylcysteine. A psychiatric assessment the day after overdose is common practice to plan any supportive interventions that might be necessary. This may include simple medical follow-up, individual therapy, group or family work or pharmacotherapy. One clear issue for this woman relates to her coping ability under adversity. The opportunity to provide supportive psychoeducation should not be missed.

Key Points

- Paracetamol overdoses are the most common overdoses with many patients not knowing the potential liver complications, including liver failure and death.
- It is always important to conduct a detailed mental state examination and consider referral for psychiatric assessment.
- Early presentation of paracetamol overdose is less complicated than late presentations.

CASE 22: FEAR OF SPIDERS

Fear history

A 20-year-old woman comes to see her general practitioner (GP) saying that a fear of spiders is causing her significant problems. When she sees a spider she becomes fearful. She sweats, shakes and her heart rate increases. She needs to get out of the room very quickly and requires family members to come and remove the spider. She cannot re-enter the room until she is certain the spider is gone. She cannot sleep in a room if she has seen a spider there and could not go on two school trips because of worries about encountering a spider.

She has been offered a job in a hotel as an apprentice domestic supervisor. She is keen to take it, but does not think she can do the job with her fears. She is also thinking of committing to a new relationship and up until now her family have helped her solve her problems. She has not revealed the extent of her difficulties to her boyfriend. She requests diazepam tablets, because her aunt uses these for her fear of aeroplanes, and believes them to be effective for phobias.

Mental state examination

When she comes in it is noticeable that she is on edge. She scans the room quickly and explains later that this was to check for spiders and that she does this routinely. Once she has done this she is relaxed and discusses her fears. She explains that they are 'irrational' and she knows that most spiders are harmless, but nevertheless experiences very intense anxiety. She has no evidence of other mental illness and no symptoms or signs of psychosis or depression.

Questions

- What do you say in reply to her request for diazepam?
- What is the treatment of choice?

ANSWER 22

1. A phobia is a persistent fear of a situation or object, with avoidance of the feared situation or object and powerful anticipatory anxiety. There is usually insight that the fear is irrational or out of kilter with the true risk of the situation.
2. Medication would not be used with spider phobia. Dependency is common with benzodiazepines.

The treatment of choice for spider phobia is cognitive behaviour therapy (CBT). This involves desensitization where exposure leads to habituation. A hierarchy of feared situations is built up, and client and therapist work their way through this hierarchy. This may, for example, begin with pictures, plastic spiders, cartoons and videos, and move on to dead and then live spiders. Different-sized spiders can be used. At first these may be in jars or Perspex boxes, then they may be put onto the table or into the therapist's hands. Many therapists will finish by putting a live spider on the table, teaching the client to cover it with a jar, sealing the jar with a card and then depositing the spider outside. The therapy can also lead to people touching live spiders, letting them run on their hands or using a 'spider hoover' to catch and deposit them outside. The end goal is usually mutually agreed and reviewed as it may change when therapy progresses.

Cognitively, the therapist may use psychoeducation explaining how humans are genetically programmed to fear certain shapes (as part of natural selection). Discussion about the purpose of fear and a systematic assessment of the dangerousness of spiders compared to other creatures (bees, wasps, rats, etc.) can help in the appraisal of threat. Personification of the spider as vulnerable (as opposed to threatening) and an understanding of how the human mind automatically interprets the body language of a spider as threatening can all help. A rational understanding of changes in fear after habituation goes hand in hand with the behavioural strategies and desensitization. Finally, the woman's memories of not coping in the presence of spiders need to be replaced through therapy and supplemented with many new experiences of coping. Much can be done in sessions, but homework also allows the client to see that he or she can cope on his or her own without help. The therapy should provide plenty of healthy experiences of coping with spiders that establish confidence.

Key Points

- Spider phobia is common.
- Benzodiazepines can lead to dependence and are not usually used in most phobias.
- Cognitive behaviour therapy is the treatment of choice.

CASE 23: DÉJÀ VU AND AMNESIA

History

A 32-year-old man presents with a several-month history of strange experiences. He occasionally has a strange metallic taste sensation, which may last for a few seconds up to about a minute. He then has experiences that are difficult to describe. He imagines it is a bit like an out-of-body experience. There are times he has a feeling that everything around him is a repeat but at other times even familiar people and features completely baffle him. After some minutes he is himself again but is often slightly disorientated and is often told that he has behaved rather oddly, for example, repeating automatic actions such as lip smacking. He himself has no memory of this. There is a sense of something having been lost but he is not quite sure what. These episodes are increasing in frequency and his behaviour is becoming more strange during them, which is the reason for seeking help now. Another feature that has worried him is that recently he has experienced auditory hallucinations. The hallucination does not last long, but is frightening. He has now become aware that the metallic taste and auditory hallucination precede the episodes and behaviours he cannot remember. He has not been witnessed collapsing or having any tonic- or clonic-type body movements. Over the last few months he has also had quite severe headaches, but these do not coincide with the episodes described earlier.

There is no previous medical history of note, and he has not recently experienced any trauma. He has no family history of psychotic experiences or seizures. He is not on any medication of any sort.

Mental state examination and physical examination

He is well presented and neither physical nor mental state examination reveal any abnormalities.

Questions

- What is the most likely explanation in this case?
- What is the differential diagnosis?
- What investigation is likely to be the most useful?

ANSWER 23

The most likely explanation is complex partial seizures of temporal lobe epilepsy (TLE). The features of seizures beginning in the temporal lobe vary from patient to patient in length and intensity but certain patterns are common. These auras are called *simple partial seizures* and occur in about three-quarters of people with TLE. They occur while consciousness is maintained. There may be a mixture of different feelings, emotions, thoughts and experiences, which may be familiar (sense of déjà vu) or completely foreign (*jamais vu*). Hallucinations of voices, music, people, smells or tastes may occur. A simple seizure or aura can evolve to more complex or generalized seizures, where consciousness is impaired. Auras may last for just a few seconds, or may continue as long as a minute or two. If they spread to local areas in the temporal lobes they become complex partial seizures. About 40% to 80% of people with TLE perform repetitive, automatic movements (called automatisms), such as lip smacking and rubbing the hands together. Some people have only simple partial seizures and never have a change in consciousness. In about 60% of people with TLE, the seizures spread leading to a grand mal seizure. After the complex partial seizure or secondarily generalized seizure, patients are often confused for several minutes and then gradually recover.

! Differential diagnosis

- There are several other possible things to consider in differential diagnosis. Consider absence seizures. These have classic three per second spike and wave patterns on EEG. They are shorter, have no aura, no post-ictal confusion and are not associated with complex automatisms.
- Frontal lobe complex partial seizures appear in clusters of brief seizures with abrupt onset and ending. There is a minimal post-ictal state. They may cause behavioural changes with vocalizations and complex motor and sometimes sexual automatisms. In differentiating from TLE, there may need to be EEG localization.
- Panic attacks can present in strange ways and need to be considered.
- Occipital lobe epilepsy may spread to the temporal lobe and be clinically indistinguishable from a temporal lobe seizure.

The temporal lobes are the most common locations for the origin of partial seizures, which start in one localized area. TLE can start at almost any age. Some follow a head injury or an infection that affects the brain, such as meningitis, but for the vast majority the cause is unknown. There may also be other underlying causes such as a tumour or vascular malformation. EEG can confirm the diagnosis but false negatives are common. Magnetic resonance imaging can help in localizing seizure focus.

Information and individual and family support to adjust are helpful. Medication is usually required to treat the epilepsy and the majority do well on the following drugs: carbamazepine, sodium valproate, topiramate, lamotrigine and oxcarbazepine. Surgery is an option for intractable epilepsy.

Key Points

- TLE may masquerade as psychosis or severe anxiety.
- Episodic illness should arouse strong suspicion of TLE.

CASE 24: SELF-HARMING, SUBSTANCE MISUSE AND VOLATILE RELATIONSHIPS

History

A 19-year-old woman with a 6-year history of self-harm attends the emergency department. Her self-harm is usually in the form of cutting, but every few weeks when she feels things are getting on top of her, she takes an overdose. The overdoses are usually impulsive and precipitated by a row with her boyfriend or mother. The relationship with the boyfriend is volatile and the police have been called out on more than one occasion when things have become heated and violent. The woman has alleged domestic violence but then retracts her allegations and the police have not taken any action against her boyfriend. There is also a long history of substance misuse, usually alcohol but she has also dabbled in all sorts of illegal substances. When under the influence she has had unprotected sex with men other than her boyfriend and has become pregnant on two occasions. Both times she chose to end the pregnancy feeling that if she did not her boyfriend would leave her. After each termination she had a period when she described herself as 'constantly suicidal'.

Mental state examination

Her eye contact is fleeting. She is distraught and shouting that she just wants to be left alone so that she can kill herself. She is verbally abusive and threatening violence if she is not given what she wants. She is irritable and agitated. She is unkempt and looks like she has recently been in a fight. Her speech is rapid but coherent. Objectively her mood is labile and subjectively she says that she is depressed and life is not worth living. She says she is suicidal and wants to kill herself. She is angry as she feels she is being thwarted in this. She says there is no point in living especially as her boyfriend has broken up with her. There is no evidence of any psychotic features and she is orientated in time, place and person.

> **! Personality disorder**
>
> People with personality disorders have experiences and behaviour that are markedly outside their societal norms. This demonstrates itself in enduring ways, impacting upon relationships, interpersonal functioning, emotion regulation, affective responses, impulse control and attributions about self and others.

Questions

- Given the definition of a personality disorder above, does this person have a personality disorder?
- What is the differential diagnosis?

ANSWER 24

The differential diagnosis is acute intoxication (alcohol/drugs), depression or emotionally unstable personality disorder (EUPD). The most likely primary diagnosis is EUPD. An alternative way of conceptualizing this involves the use of a multi-axial formulation that considers not only diagnosis but psychosocial factors and development. It includes an understanding of early life experiences and maladaptive coping and care seeking, as well as any organic or intellectual factors. The rich explanatory power of multi-axial classification systems makes them helpful for designing interventions. Very stressful or chaotic childhoods are commonly reported (e.g. physical and sexual abuse, neglect, hostile conflict and early parental loss or separation). This often means that the features leading to the presentation are long-standing so long-term therapeutic interventions may be helpful. Multi-axial systems used in adulthood and childhood are slightly different (see Case 78).

! Multi-axial classification (*Diagnostic and Statistical Manual of Mental Disorders*)

- Axis 1: Clinical disorder
- Axis 2: Personality and intellectual
- Axis 3: Medical or physical condition
- Axis 4: Psychosocial and environmental
- Axis 5: Global functioning

This is slightly different from the multi-axial classification used in childhood (see Case 78)

The first step in management involves calming her down so a proper assessment of such factors can take place. A risk assessment is crucial because her safety is a concern. The social support available will need exploration. Even if she is not actively suicidal, admission may be unavoidable as there is a risk that she could harm herself in this volatile state.

EUPD is a condition characterized by impulsive actions, rapidly shifting moods, and chaotic relationships. There are two types (impulsive and borderline). With both of these there is

- *Impulsivity* without thought of the consequences (e.g. unprotected sex or dangerous substance abuse)
- *Lack of self-control* with outbursts of intense anger or violence

The impulsive type is characterized by emotional instability and an inability to control impulses, with episodes of threatening behaviour and violence occurring particularly in response to criticism by others.

The borderline type is also characterized by emotional instability. People with this type of personality disorder may experience severe doubts about their self-image, aims and sexual preferences that cause upset and distress. It is common to experience a strong and debilitating sense of emptiness and this can lead to self-harm and suicide threats. They are liable to become involved in intense but unstable relationships with regular emotional crises. Completed suicide occurs in around 8%–10% of individuals with this disorder, and self-mutilation acts (e.g. cutting or burning) and suicide threats and attempts are very common. Recurrent job losses and broken marriages are common.

Co-morbidity with mood disorders, substance misuse, eating disorders (usually bulimia) or posttraumatic stress disorder (PTSD) is common. This disorder is more frequent in females than males.

Emotional instability and impulsivity are very common in adolescents, but most adolescents grow out of this behaviour. Personality disorder diagnoses are not made in adolescence because of the ongoing development of personality and the stigmatizing nature of the diagnosis. It should therefore only be carefully and cautiously applied. This disorder, like all personality disorders, is usually worse in the young adult years and gradually decreases with age. Into the 30s and beyond, the majority of individuals have attained greater stability in their relationships and working lives.

Key Points

- The diagnosis of personality disorder requires detailed longitudinal history and should not be made on the basis of one interview.
- This disorder often presents through self-harm and suicidal threats, but impulsive behaviour is common across various spheres of life.
- Individuals with this disorder have often had chaotic childhoods and have inappropriate social supports and coping mechanisms. Interventions are best directed towards remedying these limitations rather than with pharmacotherapy.

CASE 25: MY HUSBAND WON'T LET ME GO OUT

History

A 23-year-old woman comes to see the general practitioner with her mother. She has been married for 4 years. Her mother has brought her because she was in two minds about whether to come. She is worried that it may make the problem worse. The general practitioner (GP) realizes quickly that he is going to need more than 10 minutes and has one other patient left. He sees this other patient first in another consultation suite and returns in order to give more time for the discussion. The woman is in tears when he returns and describes that she loves her husband but that he is very possessive of her, and has never been happy for her to go anywhere without him. He works on a computer during the day at a large insurance firm. Despite having trained at college in Child Care she is not currently working, mainly because her husband made it clear when they married that he wanted to be the main breadwinner and did not wish for her to work. He likes to stay in and watch television, and will usually drink a few cans of lager three or four nights a week. He does not usually drink to excess.

She stopped her hobbies such as salsa lessons and going out with friends when they started seeing each other, about 3 months before they got married. He used to accuse her of flirting if he ever saw her laughing or smiling with any other man and she began to restrict who she spoke to as a means of avoiding this. She explains that about 6 months ago her best friend, whom he never really liked, began encouraging her to go out with a group of four old school friends who meet at a line dancing group and go for a drink and meal afterwards. Her husband was not keen, but let her go. When she returned he was very suspicious and asked her numerous questions about what she had been doing and whether she spoke to any other men. She considered not going any more, but with the support of her best friend and mother, decided that she was doing no harm and that he may get used to the idea. She went on four more occasions. On each occasion when she returned he insisted on examining her underwear and was aggressive and abusive, calling her offensive names. After the most recent occasion he threw the contents of all her drawers around the bedroom and forced her onto the bed, shouting in her face. She says she has never thought of involving the police.

She does not know what to do, because she feels that if she never goes out she will feel trapped, but she cannot cope with his levels of suspicion and hostility. She thinks he needs help but does not know what to do next. The woman's mother says that she has always been a quiet girl and endorses her daughter's assertion that she has never been nor would she ever be unfaithful. The mother says that her son-in-law can be sociable and charming but has always been controlling of her daughter. He has superficial friends but no one visits the house and he does not visit anyone else so far as they are aware. He will sometimes have a drink with a work colleague on the way home, but never invites his wife and has not brought this friend home.

Questions

- What are the possible causes and diagnoses?
- What might the GP suggest happens next?
- What treatments are available?

ANSWER 25

There are a few possibilities that should go through the GP's mind. The first is that this man has an alcohol problem and that over and above the drinking his wife sees he may be secretly drinking a lot more. This would amount to alcohol dependence syndrome (see Case 20). Alcohol-induced symptoms may also include psychotic symptoms such as hallucinosis or alcoholic jealousy.

It is more likely that he has a dissocial or paranoid personality disorder.

! Paranoid personality

- Excessive sensitivity to setbacks
- Tendency to bear grudges
- Automatic tendency to see neutral events as negative
- Tendency to centre on the self/narcissism
- Recurrent unfounded suspicions of infidelity or betrayal
- Tendency to see conspiracy where there is none

If of delusional intensity, pathological jealousy could be a delusional disorder (see Case 54). This is characterized by a strongly held and persistent delusion. It is not the same as schizophrenia since it is not accompanied by all the other first-rank symptoms of schizophrenia such as thought passivity, auditory hallucinations, thought disorder and 'negative' symptoms of schizophrenia. It would be important to exclude other disorders such as psychosis, depression or an anxiety disorder, but these do not stand out from the history.

It is possible he has undiagnosed Asperger syndrome, meaning he makes serious misjudgements about the motivations of others and that this leads to misinterpretations and paranoia.

Finally, it would be important to ask about past history and physical symptoms to see if there is any change in behaviour or symptoms and signs that might lead to consideration of a physical illness such as space-occupying lesion. Again this is not a high possibility but should be considered.

What happens next is not straightforward since the man in question is unaware that his wife has visited the surgery. There are no grounds for breaking confidentiality at this point although that may change in the future. The woman should be advised that were he to become physically abusive it would be appropriate to call the police. She should be given information about any local women's refuges and any domestic violence services. A confidential anonymized discussion with social services and other partners may be helpful to explore any safeguarding issues in the context of a vulnerable adult. Enquiries as to whether any trusted male members of the family may be able to approach her husband and suggest he seeks help may also be helpful.

The woman herself may have mental health needs and these should be considered. Does she need to see a counsellor who could support her to work out a way of tackling the problem? Relate (local marriage guidance counselling) will often see individuals within a marriage in the first instance as a first step in finding solutions to such difficulties. It is possible she could find an appropriate time to suggest that they go together. While the problem is essentially his own, this shared approach may help him develop insight.

Finally, the pertinent question: 'What keeps you together as a couple?' may be helpful by promoting thoughts about whether she wishes to stay in a relationship that is currently abusive.

Key Points

- If it is possible to find a way of positively engaging people with pathological jealousy it can prevent long-term unhappiness for their victims.
- Facilitating a mechanism of support (e.g. counselling) can be crucial as it prevents isolation and allows a rational perspective to be taken outside the context of the relationship.
- Families can and should use the police if individuals are at risk.

CASE 26: INTENSELY FEARFUL HALLUCINATIONS

History

A 44-year-old man is admitted to an orthopaedics ward with a fracture of the femur following a car accident. He is treated surgically and there are no postoperative complications over the next 2 days. On the third day of the admission there is rapid change in his behaviour and he becomes verbally aggressive towards the nursing staff. He has been advised bed rest but tries to get up from his bed and is agitated. He is sweating, has tremors in both hands and is shouting at the nursing staff. The nurses try to restrain him but he resists actively. He is screaming that he can see snakes in the room and is terrified. He is disorientated and believes that he is in his office rather than in hospital. He is not able to recognize any of the doctors or nurses and becomes startled when the doctor's bleeper goes off. He has a history of heavy alcohol use over the past 15 years. He does not have any other medical or psychiatric history.

Mental state examination

His eye contact is not good. He appears distracted and looks across your shoulder and around the room. He is jittery and sweating, and is confused and disorientated. He is experiencing visual hallucinations which appear to be vivid and well formed. He is terrified apparently in response to these hallucinations. He is labile in his behaviour which changes rapidly with periods of increased agitation and restlessness when he attempts to get off the bed. He has little understanding of what is happening to him and is unable to discuss this in any meaningful way.

Physical examination

He has a blood pressure of 160/100 mm Hg and a pulse of 130 beats per minute. His oxygen saturation in air is 98%. He is febrile with a temperature of 38.4°C. He has coarse bilateral hand tremors and the extremities are cold and clammy and he is clinically dehydrated. He has palmar erythema.

Investigations

	Levels	*Reference range*
Haemoglobin	14.2 g/dL	11.7–15.7 g/dL
White blood cell count	9.5×10^9/L	$3.5–11.0 \times 10^9$/L
Mean corpuscular volume (MCV)	111 fL	80–99 fL
Sodium	128 mmol/L	135–145 mmol/L
Potassium	4.3 mmol/L	3.5–5.0 mmol/L
Urea	7.4 mmol/L	2.5–6.7 mmol/L
Creatinine	84 µmol/L	70–120 µmol/L
Alkaline phosphatase	406 IU/L	30–300 IU/L
Alkaline aminotransferase	130 IU/L	5–35 IU/L
Bilirubin	24 µmol/L	2–17 µmol/L
Albumin	23 g/L	35–50 g/L
Gamma-glutamyl transaminase	181 IU/L	11–51 IU/L
Random blood glucose	4.1 mmol/L	4.0–6.0 mmol/L

Questions

- What is the differential diagnosis?
- How would you manage this patient?

ANSWER 26

The patient is suffering from an acute confusional state, most likely delirium tremens (DT). Around 5% of patients admitted to hospital with alcohol-related problems have DT. There is a significant associated mortality at around 5%, and this is usually due to co-morbid medical illnesses like infections, electrolyte imbalance and impaired liver and kidney functions. It occurs when a patient dependent on alcohol suddenly stops or greatly reduces the alcohol intake. The typical symptoms of alcohol withdrawal are tremulousness, perceptual abnormalities like visual hallucinations that can be vivid and intense, withdrawal seizures and impairment of consciousness. Tremors develop within 6–8 hours, hallucinations within 12 hours and seizures within 24 hours of cessation of drinking alcohol. DT typically develops by 72 hours post-cessation of alcohol use but can develop anytime within the first week. The full-blown symptoms of DT include tremors of the body, clouding of consciousness and restlessness with vivid and intense visual hallucinations. Patients can also experience auditory hallucinations and paranoid delusions. Other symptoms include fever, excessive sweating, palpitations, nausea and vomiting. It may present in a sudden and dramatic way in patients admitted to hospital with a problem unrelated to alcohol abuse. The symptoms typically get worse at night. Patients can represent a difficult management problem in acute medical wards due to their unpredictable behaviour and the risk of acting out on perceptual abnormalities.

! Differential diagnosis

- Acute confusional states may be caused by infections (pneumonia, urinary tract infections, encephalitis), endocrine abnormalities (hypoglycaemia), metabolic abnormalities (electrolyte imbalance) or head injuries.
- Wernicke encephalopathy presents with a triad of ataxia, ophthalmoplegia and mental confusion.
- Alcoholic hallucinosis is a rare condition in which auditory hallucinations can occur in clear consciousness. The hallucinations can begin as simple sounds like a buzzing sound but can progress to well-formed voices. Most cases resolve within a few days and respond well to antipsychotics.

Taking an alcohol history is an important part of any admission to enable planning and prevention. Patients withdrawing from alcohol need to be monitored closely to prevent progression to DT. They should be nursed in a well-lit and safe environment. Dehydration, electrolyte and nutritional imbalance should be corrected by giving parenteral vitamins and fluids. A long-acting benzodiazepine like chlordiazepoxide 20–30 mg (up to four times a day) should be started. Chlordiazepoxide should be prescribed on a reducing regimen, reducing the dose every 2 days with a view to stopping over 7 days. Antipsychotic medication should be avoided as it is likely to reduce the seizure threshold and can precipitate withdrawal seizures. Advice about lifestyle changes can be given once the acute situation has settled. Motivational interviewing may be a helpful way to engage the patient in a non-judgemental way that can lay the foundations for future change.

Key Points

- Delirium tremens is characterized by tremulousness, withdrawal seizures and intense and vivid visual hallucinations with fluctuating consciousness.
- Immediate management involves medical care including rehydration, detoxification and sedation using benzodiazepines and parenteral vitamins.

CASE 27: FLASHBACKS AND NIGHTMARES

History

A 28-year-old single woman presents to her general practitioner and explains that she has been experiencing recurrent nightmares over the past 2 months. She was involved in a road traffic accident 4 months ago. The car that she had been driving crashed on the motorway killing a colleague who had been her passenger. She also sustained injuries which required a 2-week stay in hospital. She works as a manager in a building company and her job requires her to travel to different sites in her car. Since the accident she has been off work. She says that the nightmares are related to the accident. She is unable to get the memories of the accident out of her mind and can experience very vivid images of the events even during the day. She struggles with persistent anxiety and has poor sleep and concentration. She now stays at home most of the time and finds it difficult to travel by car, even as a passenger. Her mood and behaviour can fluctuate rapidly during the day, and she has recently started self-harming by making cuts to her forearms. She lives alone but has support from friends and family who live locally. There is no history of mental illness in the family. She has no previous psychiatric or medical history apart from a history of overdose with paracetamol 8 years ago. At that time she had split up with her boyfriend and took the overdose while intoxicated with alcohol. She is a non-smoker and has used cannabis in the past when she was at university. She does not use any drugs now. She used to drink alcohol socially but recently has started drinking every day. She says that she drinks one bottle of wine a day.

Mental state examination

She makes good eye contact. She appears to be anxious and has tremors in both hands. She is reluctant to speak about the road traffic accident and starts shouting, becoming verbally aggressive when questioned about the accident. There is no pressure of speech. She describes experiencing the accident as recurrent intrusive imagery. She feels guilty about surviving the accident and states that it would have been better if she had died instead of her colleague. She has thoughts that life is not worth living, but states that she would not commit suicide because of her family. Her mood is labile. There is no evidence of delusions or hallucinations. She has good insight into her difficulties.

Physical examination

Physical examination is unremarkable.

Questions

- What is the differential diagnosis?
- How would you investigate and manage this patient in general practice?

ANSWER 27

This woman is presenting with posttraumatic stress disorder (PTSD). There is an intense and prolonged reaction to severe trauma. Such trauma could be due to natural disasters (earthquake, floods, tsunami), accidents (road traffic accidents, fires) or serious physical harm/threat of harm (rape, torture, assault). This woman had an accident 4 months ago and has been experiencing symptoms of hyper-arousal (anxiety, insomnia) as well as recurrent and intrusive flashbacks. She has nightmares and has been avoiding situations that remind her of the accident (unable to travel in a car). These symptoms have presented within 6 months of the trauma and have been present for more than 1 month. She has a maladaptive style of coping and has been using excessive alcohol.

! Stress-related disorders – differential diagnosis

- Acute stress reaction is a transient disorder that occurs in response to a severely stressful event. It starts within a few hours of exposure and usually resolves within 2–3 days of the termination of the stress. Symptoms include those of anxiety, feeling of numbness, depersonalization, poor concentration and disorientation.
- Adjustment disorders occur when stressors are not life-threatening or out of normal human experience. Symptoms are depressive and/or those of anxiety, and they can affect behaviour. Symptoms do not usually persist for more than 6 months and resolve spontaneously with conservative management.
- Dissociative disorders, which are disruptions to awareness, perception or memory, can occur after stress. Dissociative amnesia and depersonalization are examples.
- Substance abuse: LSD users can experience flashbacks. Alcohol or drug intoxication or withdrawal can present with similar symptoms.
- Organic causes such as head injury can mimic or exacerbate symptoms of PTSD.
- Conversion disorders occur when stress is thought to be internalized and symptoms such as loss of power or sensation occur. Pseudoseizures may also occur.

Detailed history of previous traumatic experiences including the nature and duration of the current symptoms, along with a detailed mental state examination, is needed to rule out the above diagnoses. Urine drug screen helps rule out intoxication with illicit drugs. The immediate management would be to support and encourage her to talk about the traumatic event and to facilitate healthy emotional processing and coping. On account of the severity of her symptoms and the development of secondary complications like self-harm and alcohol misuse, she should be referred to specialist psychiatric services. She would benefit with input from a community psychiatric nurse (CPN) who could monitor her mental state and also offer help with practical issues. Trauma-focused psychological help in the form of cognitive behaviour therapy (CBT) or eye movement and desensitization reprocessing (EMDR) are first-line treatments. Pharmacological treatments are second-line treatments and include paroxetine or mirtazapine, which can be used in primary care, or amitriptyline or phenelzine, which can only be prescribed by mental health specialists.

Key Points

- PTSD follows an out of 'normal human experience' trauma. Characteristic symptoms include recollection, nightmares, flashbacks, avoidance of places or events reminiscent of trauma and anxiety symptoms.
- Trauma-focused psychological therapies are the treatments of choice.

CASE 28: UNSTEADY GAIT

History

A 50-year-old electrician presents to the emergency department with a 3-day history of an unsteady gait and double vision when looking to the right. He appears confused and gives a history of severe vomiting over the past 10 days with significant weight loss over the past few months. He has been abusing alcohol for 30 years and has been diagnosed with alcohol dependence. He underwent partial gastrectomy for carcinoma of the stomach 12 years ago. He has no other previous medical or psychiatric history.

Mental state examination

His eye contact is variable. He is disorientated. He has poor orientation in time and does not know where he is, but he is able to recognize his wife who accompanies him. He is drowsy, has poor concentration but is readily rousable. He scores 14/30 on the Mini Mental State Examination. A thorough mental state examination is difficult due to his condition, but he does not appear to be responding to any unseen stimuli. He has little insight into why he is here.

Physical examination

A general examination reveals bilateral pedal oedema and icterus. His blood pressure is 90/60 mm Hg and pulse is 120 beats per minute. Oxygen saturation on air is 96%. He has palmar erythema and hepatomegaly. He has nystagmus. Neurological examination reveals reduced power in both lower limbs. He has reduced sensation on pinprick and two-point discrimination in both lower limbs. Deep tendon reflex at the ankle is reduced bilaterally. He has an unsteady gait and is unable to stand without support.

Investigations

	Levels	*Reference range*
Haemoglobin	14.2 g/dL	11.7–15.7 g/dL
White blood cell count	9.5×10^9/L	$3.5–11.0 \times 10^9$/L
Mean corpuscular volume (MCV)	110 fL	80–99 fL
Sodium	129 mmol/L	135–145 mmol/L
Potassium	4.3 mmol/L	3.5–5.0 mmol/L
Urea	7.4 mmol/L	2.5–6.7 mmol/L
Creatinine	84 µmol/L	70–120 µmol/L
Alkaline phosphatase	356 IU/L	30–300 IU/L
Alkaline aminotransferase	92 IU/L	5–35 IU/L
Bilirubin	22 µmol/L	2–17 µmol/L
Albumin	29 g/L	35–50 g/L
Gamma-glutamyl transaminase	141 IU/L	11–51 IU/L
Random blood glucose	4.1 mmol/L	4.0–6.0 mmol/L

Magnetic resonance imaging (MRI) brain scan reveals bilateral symmetrical high-intensity areas in the thalamus and generalized cortical atrophy.

Questions

- What is the diagnosis?
- What complications can arise in the immediate management of this condition?
- How would you manage this patient?

ANSWER 28

This man is presenting with a triad of ataxia, nystagmus and confusion indicating a diagnosis of Wernicke encephalopathy (WE). This can present abruptly and is a medical emergency. It is important to recognize and treat the condition early as it is potentially reversible. This condition is related to thiamine deficiency. Thiamine is phosphorylated to TPP (thiamine pyrophosphate). TPP acts as co-factor for enzymes like transketolase and pyruvate dehydrogenase, which are essential for synthesis of myelin and also play a key role in brain glucose metabolism. Chronic alcohol use is an important cause of the condition as it impairs the absorption of thiamine from the gut. Other causes of WE include prolonged diarrhoea, vomiting, hyperemesis gravidarum, severe malnutrition in anorexia nervosa, prolonged intravenous feeding and carcinoma of the stomach.

Pathological lesions in WE involve mamillary bodies, thalamus, hypothalamus, medulla, pons and cerebellum. With prompt treatment the condition is reversible and greatly reduces the risk of subsequent cognitive impairment. WE is pathophysiologically related to Korsakoff syndrome (KS). Many of the cases of WE can progress to KS, which is characterized by poverty in the content of conversation and confabulation. There is enduring cognitive impairment with loss of recent memory, anterograde amnesia and the sufferer has little insight into his or her problem. In cases of established KS, the prognosis is poor with very few patients improving even with continued thiamine treatment.

! Complications of WE

- Strict bed rest is required in the acute stages of presentation. There is a risk of cardiovascular collapse. Sudden death can occur due to cardiac decompensation. In patients with signs of cardiac failure, digitilization might be needed.
- Thiamine should always be administered before carbohydrate or glucose infusion as thiamine is required for glucose metabolism, and glucose infusion can rapidly deplete the thiamine stores and further aggravate the condition.

This patient needs to be given 50 mg of thiamine intravenously, given slowly over 10 minutes due to risk of anaphylactic reaction. This should be accompanied by intramuscular (IM) injection of 50 mg of thiamine. The IM thiamine should be continued for 5 days during which the normal diet is resumed. Absorption of thiamine from the gastrointestinal tract can be inconsistent and therefore oral administration is not reliable. Injection of Pabrinex, which contains nicotinamide, riboflavine, pyridoxine and ascorbic acid along with thiamine, is often preferable to thiamine alone as this will cover the possibility of other vitamin deficiencies. The patient needs complete bed rest. Management would involve also giving consideration to the possibility of infection, dehydration and electrolyte imbalance. Oral thiamine 100 mg twice daily should be continued for 6–12 months after acute illness has resolved. Lifestyle advice and family support will be helpful.

Key Points

- WE is characterized by a triad of ataxia, nystagmus and confusion. When suspecting WE, always ensure thiamine is administered before giving glucose.
- WE may lead to Korsakoff psychosis, which is not a psychotic disorder but is a cognitive disorder with poorer cognitive prognosis.

CASE 29: THIS PAIN JUST WON'T GO AWAY

History

A 43-year-old woman has been coming to her general practitioner (GP) for 3 years with pelvic pain. She has seen two different gynaecologists in that time and has had numerous investigations, but a cause has not been identified. She comes to the surgery again with the same symptom saying that she is unable to have sex with her husband and feels a sharp pain like a bone pushing inside her almost constantly. Prior to this she had right-sided hypochondrial pain for a 2-year period and received a computed tomography (CT) scan and two ultrasounds that showed no abnormalities, before the symptoms spontaneously remitted. In her notes it shows that in her early thirties she was investigated for central chest pain and difficulty swallowing. An endoscopy, CT scan of her chest and chest X-rays were all normal. She has had irritable bowel syndrome since she was 16. She has intermittently been off work but has never been off long term and enjoys her role as a receptionist at the local hospital's patient advice and liaison service.

When you ask her today about other symptoms she indicates that she has no heavy periods although she sometimes bleeds for up to 9 days. For the last 6 months she has had intermittent palpitations, dizziness and nausea. She is asking for a sick note and a referral to the hospital, but she does not want to see either of the gynaecologists she has seen before.

A brief scan of previous investigations shows that they have been numerous and normal.

Questions

- What diagnoses go through your mind?
- What do you decide to do?

ANSWER 29

It is important not to fall into the trap of automatically dismissing this woman's symptoms. However, the history is fairly typical of somatization disorder (see Case 18). Malingering is another possibility although the fact that she enjoys her work makes this unlikely.

Somatization disorder

- Chronic single or multiple symptoms
- Symptoms occurring across different body systems
- Symptoms with no explanatory objective signs or investigations
- Psychiatric disorder, such as depression, often present
- Numerous past investigations
- Rejection of previous physicians

In essence the task of the GP is to rule out physical causes and then to seek some kind of help that will prevent long-term social, marital or occupational handicap. The key to these situations is to know when to raise alternative courses other than persistent investigation. Investigation is costly for several reasons. It engenders anxiety in the individual about possible pathology. Studies examining case notes of somatizing patients reveal very high lifetime costs to the health service often with little or no benefit.

The best timing to discuss the possibility of somatization is when a tranche of investigations have come back that are normal. It could be that the GP in this situation discusses previous results or seeks a further referral and discusses with the consultant concerned the importance of steering the woman towards alternative attributions about the nature of her symptoms. Somatization disorder is not malingering in the sense that symptoms are not feigned. Symptoms are experienced as real. If a patient is being told that there is no physical explanation for his or her symptoms it is important not to imply that the patient is in some way 'making up' the symptoms but instead, offer some explanation of where they originate from. Clinicians may explain that the body's nervous system is very complicated and that sometimes pain or other symptoms can occur when there is no physical treatable pathology. Some people experience pains or symptoms spontaneously for no known reason and some experience them where stress or factors such as poor sleep or poor diet affect nervous system function. Opening up this discourse allows the clinician to make appropriate referrals to professionals such as a clinical psychologist or liaison psychiatrist who can give support to these aspects of functioning. The focus may not be on cure, but on coping. If the woman is not receptive to such a referral an alternative pragmatic approach would be to discuss lifestyle changes, coping strategies or holistic activities such as yoga or aromatherapy that focus on general well-being, not the main symptom.

Finally screen for depression which is commonly present. If it is present appropriate treatment may help.

Key Points

- Somatization disorder should be considered if symptoms occurring across physical systems are chronic and have resulted in repeated negative investigations.
- Treat depression if present.
- Successful treatment reduces unnecessary investigations and facilitates a better quality of life.

CASE 30: CAN'T CONCENTRATE AFTER HIS DAUGHTER DIED

History

A 32-year-old man attends the general practitioner (GP) surgery because after his 18-month-old daughter died 6 months ago he has been unable to concentrate. He went back to work in an insurance firm after 2 weeks but finds it hard, and feels a strong emotional jolt every time he signs his signature. He explains that his daughter had been born with a heart defect, and that he had been the one who signed the consent form for her to have the heart operation. He cannot get it out of his mind that it was like him signing her death warrant. He feels angry with medical staff, although he says that they did nothing wrong that he knows of. She died a day after surgery when she suffered disseminated intravascular coagulation.

He has lost his appetite, his sleep is poor and he is drinking more alcohol than usual. He can concentrate at home on television programmes. He feels a general lack of energy and says that he has difficulty enjoying things any more (anhedonia). If he laughs he feels guilty. Prior to his daughter's operation he was happy, although understandably concerned about his daughter's health. He also regularly went out with friends, including five-a-side football on a Friday night followed by drinks and a meal. He could laugh and enjoy himself at this time. He has no history of depression or psychiatric or psychological problems.

His wife is low in mood but has returned to work in a human resources department of a large manufacturing firm. She values the support of her friends there and has accessed ad hoc counselling through her occupational health department.

They have one other child, a boy aged 7 who is missing his baby sister. He is cheerful much of the time but cries sometimes at night saying he misses their cuddles. He is well cared for.

Mental state examination

He is well dressed in chinos and an ironed open-necked shirt. His eye contact is good. He has no agitation or psychomotor retardation. His mood is low and he describes being tearful about once per week. His thoughts are normal in flow, speed and content. He has no thought passivity or hallucinations or delusions. He is not suicidal although he admits that life seems a bit pointless. He says he would never kill himself because he loves his son too much. He cannot see the point of going to work when his baby girl is dead, but goes to 'bring the money in'. He has insight into the fact that he is feeling this way because of 'grief'.

Questions

- What is the problem?
- How can you help?

ANSWER 30

It is important to consider the diagnosis of depression. However, this man's mental health was good prior to the death of his daughter. His current problems clearly occur in the context of bereavement, and many aspects represent appropriate responses. A diagnosis of depression may unnecessarily pathologize him at a time when he needs support. The best thing to do at this point is to record the symptoms of depression and monitor them once you have provided bereavement support. A risk assessment would need to be carried out to make sure that he poses no risk to himself. There are no early indications of suicidal ideation in his case.

Normal bereavement can include low mood, sleep disturbance and tearfulness. Often such symptoms abate with time. This varies but about four-fifths will experience improvements in these symptoms 4 months post bereavement. Theorists regard that certain emotions are seen commonly in bereavement, which include numbness of emotion or even denial that the event has occurred. Yearning and distress, sadness, preoccupation with the dead person, reminiscing, acceptance and readjustment can all be part of the spectrum of the bereavement response evolving over time. Experiences of 'what if' or 'if only' are common. It should be remembered that 'loss' never disappears, memories can elicit both positive feelings and regret for years. Visions of the person who has died can occur, and these are usually recognized as not 'real' and as such are pseudohallucinations (true hallucinations are perceived as indistinguishable from actual perceptions). They usually disappear with time.

Pathological grief is not a clearly defined concept. It has a lengthy and varied literature which reflects the difficulty of attributing a 'norm' to a process determined by different individuals' personalities and coping resources. It refers to situations where a person's grieving process is significantly hampered in some way and affects his or her functioning beyond an expected range. The most common example would be where it is prolonged and severe. This man's grief has lasted 6 months thus far and could not be described as pathological. This label should only be applied if the clinician is clear that using such a label may help.

The best thing to do in this situation is to make sure that this man has good support. Ask about friends and family and what his sources of support are. Bereavement support can come from many different places determined by the individual's preferences. It may come from religious advisors, family, friends, third-sector counsellors (e.g. Cruse Bereavement Care), funeral director services or through general practice counsellors. Some areas run bereavement groups which, although often focused on the needs of children, also provide support to parents and carers. The needs and well-being of this man's wife and children should also be considered. Follow-up is necessary to monitor whether the situation improves. If it does not, a referral to a psychologist or local bereavement service would be appropriate.

Key Points

- Bereavement is not an abnormal experience.
- Family members can benefit from support after bereavement. This varies enormously depending on personal preference.

CASE 31: SOMETHING'S NOT QUITE RIGHT

History

A 24-year-old man's parents bring him to see you. Up until a few months ago he seemed to be doing well and there were no concerns. He was in the second year of his PhD, but then apparently quite suddenly lost interest in his academic work and also stopped socializing with his friends. He returned to live at home and has been increasingly more withdrawn at home. He is speaking less and less and is becoming apathetic and rarely shows any emotion or engagement with anyone including his family members with whom he had been reasonably close. When asked how he is, the man insists he is fine and he cannot understand his parents' concern. When asked about what they think is wrong, his parents cannot say what concerns them, but they are sure something is not right.

Mental state examination

His eye contact is variable and when he does make eye contact it is fixed but there is no sense of rapport with you. He is a polite and reasonably cooperative man. He does not appear anxious or agitated but appears rather flat in affect. He seems slightly detached from his parents and does not look at them. His speech appears normal, but he does at times struggle to answer even quite basic questions and his responses are short. He describes his mood as 'fine' and denies any self-harm ideation. He does not look depressed but seems detached and in a world of his own. He denies any hallucinations or delusions. There is no evidence of any thought disorder, although he says very little so this is difficult to elicit. He is orientated in time, place and person. His serial sevens testing is poor, but his parents say he has never been good at mathematics.

You then call (with his consent) his university tutor who reports that a few months prior to him leaving university and returning home, it was brought to the tutor's attention by his peers that there had been episodes of strange and erratic behaviour. By the time the university health service saw him, the episodes seemed to have settled, but it was suggested he would benefit from a break.

Questions

- What is the differential diagnosis?
- How would you manage this case?

ANSWER 31

The man needs to be assessed and he will need to be seen alone. If he has capacity, his consent is required to share information about his care with his parents. You will need to ask about any changes in mood, any experience of perceptual abnormality, any evidence of delusions and any changes in behaviour. A risk assessment is also needed.

The differential diagnoses will include depression, substance misuse, schizophrenia presenting with negative symptoms, autism spectrum disorder (extremely unlikely as onset appears to be recent and autism spectrum disorder would have displayed features from before age 3) and possible organic causes.

The most likely diagnoses are depression or schizophrenia. This man appears to be presenting with the negative symptoms of schizophrenia, but it is important not to jump too quickly to conclusions as making this diagnosis has a number of weighty implications for this man and his family. Make sure that other possibilities are excluded.

! Negative symptoms and signs of schizophrenia

- Avolition and low energy – the person tends to sit around and sleep much more than normal, lacks interest in life and has poor motivation.
- Affective flattening – a blank, blunted facial expression or less lively facial movements, flat voice (lack of normal intonations and variance) or physical movements and poverty of emotional expression compared to before.
- Alogia describes poverty of speech.
- Interest in others is reduced.
- Inability to make friends or keep friends.
- Social isolation.
- Poor self-care.
- Catatonia can present in a number of ways with profound effects on movement and activity. There may be an apparent unawareness of the environment, near total absence of motion and speech, aimless body movements and bizarre postures.

Although there are no tests that can diagnose schizophrenia, simple blood and urine tests can rule out other medical causes of symptoms. Brain imaging studies, such as magnetic resonance imaging or a computed tomography scan, can exclude other rare problems such as space-occupying lesions. A thorough history and blood screen could exclude any missed systemic illness such as anaemia or hypothyroidism.

The management of this man would depend on the final diagnosis. Initial treatment may focus on psychosocial interventions including psychoeducation, activity scheduling, family therapy and cognitive behaviour therapy. Other aspects of treatment include the development of coping strategies and helping him function the best he can whatever the symptoms are. Depression would warrant antidepressants, and a diagnosis of schizophrenia would involve treatment with antipsychotic medication, although compliance may be an issue as the man does not believe he is unwell. Psychosocial interventions would allow a period of monitoring before deciding on medication. Antipsychotics appear less effective in reducing negative symptoms than positive ones. Educating and supporting the family are also important components of care. It is very important that patients stay in treatment even after recovery. Four out of five patients who stop taking their medication after a first episode of schizophrenia will have a relapse. Relapse prevention work is therefore a key part of any treatment programme.

Key Points

- Antipsychotic medication is less effective for the negative symptoms of schizophrenia; only with clozapine is there good evidence of significant effects on negative symptoms.
- Educating and supporting the family are key components of care.

CASE 32: TRICYCLIC ANTIDEPRESSANT OVERDOSE

History

A 20-year-old law student attends the emergency department with her parents after having taken an overdose of her mother's antidepressant medication. She had a row earlier in the day with her parents about her mobile phone bill. She says that, in a fit of anger, she locked herself in the bathroom and swallowed a fistful of pills. She is carrying the bottle labelled 'dothiepin 75 mg', which may have contained as many as 28 tablets. She is very remorseful about the attempt and says it was impulsive. She has apologized to her parents and has come to the emergency department at their insistence. She says she feels fine and reports no symptoms apart from a slight pain in her abdomen. She reports feeling drowsy and would like to go home to 'sleep it off'. There is no past history of any mental illness though her father says that she has always been a 'moody girl' and has periods where she is very low, tired and feeling worthless about herself. At other times, she can be vivacious, spending a lot of money, full of confidence and brimming with ideas.

Mental state examination

She appears drowsy and her speech is slurred. She is constantly licking her lips and sipping water from a bottle. Her mood is euthymic. She expresses remorse and denies any ideas of self-harm. There are no psychotic symptoms. She appears a little disorientated, getting the time and date wrong, but there is no evidence of gross cognitive abnormality. There is no evidence of any other psychopathology. She is willing to be examined but refuses to be admitted.

Physical examination

She appears flushed and warm to touch. Her temperature is 38°C. Her pulse is 110 beats per minute and irregular and blood pressure is 98/64 mm Hg. Her pupils are dilated. There are no focal signs on central nervous system (CNS) examination. Abdominal examination reveals a distended bladder.

Question

- How will you manage this patient?

ANSWER 32

This woman is claiming to be fine, but she is presenting with an overdose of tricyclic antidepressants (TCAs), which can potentially be fatal and is therefore a medical emergency. She needs to be observed and investigated in a medical assessment unit for at least 6–8 hours as symptoms may commence only 2 hours after the overdose with major complications occurring typically within the first 6 hours. These can be very serious and require treatment in an intensive care unit (ICU). If she lacks the capacity to refuse treatment, she may need to be assessed and treated against her will using the appropriate legislation – Mental Capacity Act in England and Wales. This assessment will need to be carried out by the emergency department consultant.

She is presenting with an anticholinergic syndrome – 'Blind as a bat, Red as a beet, Hot as a hare, Dry as a bone, Mad as a hatter'. However, toxic effects are also due to alpha-adrenergic blockade (vasodilation, hypotension and cardiogenic shock), reuptake inhibition of noradrenaline and serotonin (tachycardia and seizures) and sodium channel blockade (slow depolarization of the action potential and prolonged PR, QRS and QT intervals). Impaired cardiac conduction may lead to heart block, unstable ventricular arrhythmias or asystole. Direct depression of myocardial contractility may also be seen.

Investigations

- Toxicology screen – to rule out co-ingestion of other substances. The regional toxicology laboratory or TOXBASE may offer specific advice.
- Blood tests – including complete blood count (CBC), urea and electrolytes (hypokalaemia often seen), renal function tests (impaired renal function prolongs toxicity as TCAs are excreted by the kidneys).
- Arterial blood gases are vital as TCA toxicity leads to mixed acidosis due to respiratory depression and hypotension secondary to myocardial depression and peripheral vasodilation. The acidosis in turn decreases protein binding and increases plasma levels of free drug.
- Electrocardiogram (ECG) has diagnostic and prognostic significance – limb lead QRS >160 milliseconds and R wave >3 mm in lead aVR are associated with increased risk of seizures and ventricular arrhythmias and are better predictors than plasma TCA levels.

Securing ABC (airway, breathing and circulation) is necessary. Early gastric decontamination using activated charcoal should be considered if patient presents within the first hour or two of ingestion. Reversing acidosis with sodium bicarbonate when pH <7.1 is vital. Antiarrhythmics should be avoided. Hypoxia, hypotension and hypokalaemia should be corrected while symptomatic treatment should be instituted for seizures (benzodiazepines) and urinary retention (catheter). Prolonged resuscitation is known to be successful in patients with cardiac arrest. She should be monitored for at least 24 hours after ECG returns to normal. Psychiatric assessment is essential prior to discharge to assess further risk of self-harm. She has periodic fluctuations of mood, which should arouse suspicion of bipolar disorder or cyclothymic disorder (periods of depressive symptoms alternating with hypomanic symptoms for >2 years not meeting criteria for depression or bipolar disorder). Selective serotonin reuptake inhibitors (SSRIs) are safer than TCAs should she ever need an antidepressant.

Key Points

- TCA overdose is a serious medical emergency needing cardiac monitoring.
- Appropriate legal frameworks should be used to treat patients lacking the capacity to refuse treatment.
- SSRIs are safer than TCAs in overdose.

CASE 33: SUICIDAL RISK ASSESSMENT

History

A 29-year-old man presents with his sixth deliberate self-harm episode in 4 months. He has made four attempts to hang himself (including this one), jumped out of a building and thrown himself in front of traffic. There is no evidence of any injury. He was brought to the emergency department as he tried to hang himself outside his girlfriend's house. Each hanging attempt has been triggered by an argument with his estranged girlfriend. He wants to ensure that she is aware of what he is doing and the extent to which he is suffering because of her behaviour. There is some evidence that the relationship was previously volatile. He has been charged with domestic violence in the past, but the charges were subsequently dropped as she withdrew her complaint. There is no suicide note and he has made no efforts to settle any of his affairs. He does not have any strong ties to anyone in particular and most of his relationships tend to be fairly transitory as he ends up falling out with people. He is quite charming to the female nurses and slightly hostile with the male charge nurse. However, on finding out that he has to wait to be assessed, he becomes very angry and starts threatening violence.

Questions

- What are the factors associated with completed suicide?
- What are the key questions that should be asked in an assessment of risk?

ANSWER 33

Most self-harm episodes do not result in suicide, but the risks are increased if there is co-morbidity with a mental illness. Psychiatric diagnoses classically associated with completed suicide include major mood disorders, schizophrenia and addiction disorders. Two or more psychiatric disorders may interact to greatly increase the risk of suicide compared to a level that either diagnosis alone might carry, especially alcohol problems and depression. Suicide notes and planned suicides without any intention of being discovered (e.g. not disclosing the attempt to anyone) are particularly worrying. Males are more likely to use violent methods which may mean that impulsive attempts are more likely to be fatal. Firearm availability is an independent suicide risk factor. Well-identified demographic and biopsychosocial risk factors consistently associated with completed suicide in the general population include male gender, older age, white race, widowed status, poor health (especially if painful serious illness is present) and lack of social support. Patients with previous serious attempts, a family history of completed suicide, history of drug/alcohol dependence, history of psychiatric illness, history of chronic or painful physical conditions and emotional feelings of hopelessness are also at significantly higher risk of killing themselves. In addition the severity of previous attempts in a patient's life history is predictive of future suicide risk. The two personality disorders most frequently associated with completed suicide are emotionally unstable personality disorder (EUPD) and dissocial personality disorder (DPD). This man may have DPD given the history and may be at risk until the issues relating to the current girlfriend are resolved.

The woman concerned is also at risk from him. A risk assessment involves assessing risk to others as well as self as a result of the patient's mental state. The following are fairly standard screening questions.

Useful questions in assessment of risk of harm to self

1. Have you ever felt that life is not worth living?
    - How long do those feelings last?
    - Do they come and go or are they there all the time?
    - Can you manage the feelings?
2. Have you thought about acting on the feelings?
3. Have you made any plans?
    - How close have you come to acting on the thoughts?
    - What stopped you doing anything?
    - Have you tried anything before?
    - How can I trust that you will be able to keep yourself safe?
4. Do you feel unsafe?

If the feelings of self-harm are pervasive and there is an urge to act on them and plans have been made, the risk is high.

Make sure that there is an assessment of risk of potential harm to others (see Case 42) and risk of self-neglect. If there is any potential risk of him harming his girlfriend it is likely that confidentiality will need to be breached. She and/or the police may need to be informed to ensure her safety. Discuss and document these risks and decisions.

Key Points

- Most people who present with self-harm do not go on to commit suicide; however, one presentation of self-harm increases the likelihood of further attempts.
- Risk assessment is a key skill that all doctors need to be able to undertake.
- A complete risk assessment would also include risk to others (including adults and children, and risk of self-neglect or vulnerability to exploitation).
- Even patients who frustrate you or make you angry need a proper risk assessment.

CASE 34: SUSPICIOUS AND JERKY MOVEMENTS

A 53-year-old supply teacher attends the psychiatric outpatient clinic with his wife. His wife says that his personality has 'changed completely' over the past 2 years. He has become increasingly suspicious and cantankerous. He often misplaces objects and then accuses her of stealing from him and has made similar accusations against close friends. Previously a placid person, he has now become irritable and aggressive. She feels that his 'mood swings' are now becoming intolerable. However, he says that his wife is making an 'unnecessary fuss'. He acknowledges being a 'bit low' after taking premature retirement 2 years ago, but does not feel that there is anything really wrong with him. He appears twitchy, displaying sudden 'jerky' movements of his arms and neck. He dismisses them as 'nervous tics'. His wife, however, feels that he is getting clumsy, dropping things and occasionally even stumbling.

There is no previous psychiatric history although he says he took premature retirement due to stress. There is no past medical history of note. His father died at the age of 60 following a 'nervous breakdown' in his final years but he cannot provide you with any more details. There is no other significant family history. The couple has a son, 30, and a daughter, 25, who live close by. They live in their own home.

Mental state examination

He is a tall, thin gentleman, who establishes a good rapport. His speech appears a little slurred at times but is coherent and relevant. He displays sudden jerky movements of his arms, shoulder and neck. There is no evidence of thought disorder. He is convinced that his wife and his friends have stolen money and a few of his personal objects. He acknowledges that there is no obvious motive but yet remains convinced about this. He appears low in mood but does not have any ideas of self-harm or suicide. He has little insight into his symptoms and blames it all on 'stress'. On cognitive examination, he appears a little confused about the date and time and is rather clumsy on motor tasks such as writing. Mini Mental State Examination reveals a score of 23/30 with losses on tasks of orientation (three points), tasks of concentration (two points), three-object recall (one point) and construction (one point).

Questions

- What is the differential diagnosis?
- What investigations are indicated?
- How will you manage this patient?

ANSWER 34

Pre-senile onset of cognitive, emotional and behavioural changes associated with movement disorder, in the presence of a family history, should arouse strong suspicion of the progressive degenerative disorder, Huntington disease (HD). The disease usually presents in the fourth or fifth decade, often presenting with psychiatric symptoms, most commonly personality changes, emotional disturbance and paranoia. Paranoid ideas of reference with frank delusions of persecution may be the earliest symptoms often associated with depression and anxiety. Behavioural agitation, often associated with aggression and violence, may be seen independently of choreiform movement disorder. Choreiform movements are regular, uncontrollable, random, brief muscle jerks and movements. These are different from athetoid movements, which involve writhing and twisting movements. Choreiform movements may initially be very mild and may go unnoticed for years but become florid and disabling as the disease progresses. Insidious cognitive impairment ultimately leads to severe dementia. Initially, the clinical picture resembles paranoid schizophrenia. Other psychiatric differential diagnoses include psychotic depression, bipolar disorder or schizoaffective disorder. Other causes of dementia such as Alzheimer's disease, vascular dementia, Wilson's disease, Parkinson's disease and neuroacanthocytosis also need to be considered as do other conditions such as multiple sclerosis, systemic lupus erythematosus (SLE), neurosyphilis and drug-induced cerebellar disorder.

A high index of clinical suspicion is needed to make the correct diagnosis as up to a third of cases are wrongly labelled as schizophrenia. Computed tomography (CT) and magnetic resonance imaging (MRI) brain scans reveal dilated ventricles with atrophy of the caudate nuclei and are therefore indicated in all first-time presentations of psychosis. Genetic testing is diagnostic with the identification of multiple cytosine/adenine/guanine (CAG) repeats on the short arm of chromosome 4. The normal gene shows 11–34 repeats while in HD 37–120 repeats are seen. Pre-test genetic counselling is vital as the diagnosis of the disease has implications for the patient's children with a strong likelihood (50%) of one of them being affected. It is autosomal dominant.

! Prevalance of co-morbid psychiatric symptoms

Co-morbid psychiatric symptoms (Van Duijn et al., 2007)	Prevalence
Depression, anxiety, irritability or apathy	Between 33% and 76%
Obsessions and compulsions	Between 10% and 50%
Psychosis	Up to 10%

Note: Van Duijn E, Kingma EM, Van der Mast RC. 2007. Psychopathology in verified Huntington's disease gene carriers. *Journal of Neuropsychiatry and Clinical Neurosciences* 19, 441–448.

The disease is progressive and incurable with treatment directed towards palliation of symptoms. Mean survival time is 15–18 years. Psychotic symptoms such as agitation, delusions and hallucinations and movement disorders can be treated with atypical (clozapine) or typical (haloperidol) antipsychotic medication and tranquillizers such as clonazepam. Depressive episodes usually respond to selective serotonin reuptake inhibiting antidepressants such as fluoxetine or sertraline. Manic features may need a mood stabilizer (e.g. lithium) in addition to antipsychotic medication. Obsessive rituals may need treatment with anti-obsessional agents (e.g. fluoxetine). Speech therapy for dysarthria, physiotherapy for muscle rigidity and occupational therapy to maintain and enhance activities of daily living are indicated. Support for carers and signposting to support organizations such as the Huntington's Disease Association is helpful. Referral to social services is necessary to organize community care packages, home adaptation or nursing home care.

Key Points

- HD can often be misdiagnosed as schizophrenia or mood disorder and therefore CT/MRI scans are indicated in first presentations of psychosis.
- Management involves genetic counselling and symptomatic treatment.

CASE 35: MY NOSE IS TOO BIG AND UGLY

History

A 26-year-old woman presents saying she needs referral to a plastic surgeon as her nose is too large. She feels that people constantly comment on her nose, behind her back. She feels her facial disfigurement has prevented her from developing positive relationships as she lacks confidence and never believes friends when they try to reassure her that her nose is fine. She rarely goes out as she is convinced that everyone stares at her and talks about her. She recently gave up her job as she was constantly late because it took her so long to apply her makeup to hide the disfigurement. She was also reluctant to move from the office to a receptionist role as she did not want to have to see people.

Mental state examination

Her appearance is healthy and there is no discernible abnormality with her nose in shape or size. The woman presents as affable and communicative. She is however inclined to hide her face and especially her nose by using a leaflet even though she is wearing a floppy hat which covers most of her face. Her eye contact is variable. She appears somewhat nervous and her speech is rapid but only when she is talking about her nose. She does not describe herself as low in mood and does not appear depressed. She does not have active self-harm ideation, and there is no evidence of psychosis.

Questions

- What is the diagnosis?
- What are the treatment options?

ANSWER 35

This woman has body dysmorphic disorder (BDD). She is preoccupied with a defect in her appearance that is imagined. For it to be a disorder it must lead to impairment in social or occupational functioning, and cause significant distress. The individual's symptoms must not be better accounted for by another disorder, for example, thinking he or she is fat in the context of an eating disorder, or a depressive delusion. The defect is not recognized by other people. This dislike of the defect is more than the usual negative feelings that most people have about the way they look from time to time, as it significantly impacts on functioning, especially socially. The beliefs usually represent overvalued ideas, although occasionally when insight is absent the beliefs may be delusional in quality. In this case it is important to explore co-morbidities. Co-morbidity with other psychiatric disorders is common with three-quarters of people with BDD, in that they may have major depressive disorder, social phobia or obsessive-compulsive disorder (OCD) at some point. It has been suggested that individuals with BDD are more likely to have avoidant personality disorder or dependent personality disorder which conforms to the introverted, shy and neurotic traits usually found in individuals with the disorder. BDD is sometimes called *dysmorphophobia* and is one of the hypochondriacal disorders.

Common symptoms of BDD

There are preoccupations and ruminations about a perceived defect in appearance, which sometimes lead to obsessive or compulsive behaviours. Such behaviours might include regular checking of the relevant body part or checking in the mirror, intense avoidance of mirrors or images of themselves, attempts to hide the area of concern with makeup and clothing and prolonged grooming. All of these would be to an intense degree. Some will withdraw from family or social life, becoming intensely self-conscious, and they often develop low self-esteem. In some instances mental health symptoms become more severe. Self-consciousness may become paranoia. Low mood and low self-esteem may develop into clinical depression and/or thoughts of self-harm. These persons may seek regular reassurance from those close to them, regularly comparing themselves to others. Relationships and work can suffer, and it may lead to major depression, generalized anxiety or alcohol or drug abuse.

Many individuals with BDD repeatedly seek treatment from doctors as they attempt to correct the perceived 'disfigurement'. Surgery is unlikely to help as the patient is rarely satisfied given that his or her concerns do not relate to genuine abnormal features. The overvalued ideas about disfigurement often remain or subtly alter, leading to ongoing or additional concerns. They usually accept psychiatric or psychological help reluctantly. It is a difficult disorder to treat. Psychodynamic approaches to therapy have not proven to be effective, but there has been some success with cognitive behaviour therapy (CBT). Selective serotonin reuptake inhibitors may help if there is a strong depressive component or features of OCD, but it would ideally be used alongside CBT.

Key Points

- BDD is a difficult disorder to treat and psychological treatments are usually reluctantly accepted.
- CBT is the treatment of choice.

CASE 36: CAN I TREAT HER AGAINST HER WILL?

History

A 38-year-old woman presents to the emergency department (ED) having taken an overdose some 6 hours ago. She is refusing to give consent for her blood to be taken for tests. She is also shouting 'you're not going to pump my stomach'. You are told that the psychiatrist should be called so that she can be detained against her will to enable you to take blood and enforce treatment. (In this case the patient is in England where the Mental Health Act (MHA) applies.)

She took the overdose after finding out that her husband of 15 years is leaving her. The overdose was impulsive. She wrote no note. She has three children who were in the house at the time of the overdose. She is adamant that there is no point in living, given she has been betrayed by her husband. She is sure her family will look after her children. You look up a handbook describing the Mental Health Act – (applicable in England and Wales), which outlines the main sections as presented.

! Main sections of the Mental Health Act (England and Wales)

- Section 2: An assessment order, which allows compulsory detention for 28 days.
- Section 3: A treatment order, which allows detention for 6 months.
- Section 4: An order that can be applied by a single clinician to admit a patient while arrangements are made for further assessment. Detention is for up to 72 hours.
- Section 5(2): An order that allows detention of existing inpatients for 72 hours.

Questions

- What is the role of the psychiatrist in this case?
- What are the key issues that need clarification?

ANSWER 36

Good practice involves treating patients obtaining appropriate informed consent. In this case it would be important to assess her capacity to consent to investigation and treatment but failing the capacity test does not require or necessarily imply a psychiatric diagnosis. Although this woman is unlikely to have a mental illness, her acute distress might make her temporarily incompetent from the point of view of capacity. Her capacity to refuse treatment should initially be assessed by the ED doctor and if capacity is felt to be lacking she can be treated against her will using appropriate legislation for e.g. Mental Capacity Act in England and Wales.

If the patient is deemed to have capacity but continues to refuse tests and/or treatment, she cannot be forced to accept treatment. However it is important to keep a dialogue going with her and to enlist the help of someone she trusts to try and persuade her to change her mind. In severe emergencies where treatment for life-threatening conditions is necessary without consent (e.g. an unconscious patient), the treating team should ensure that treatments are in the best interests of the patient, and where possible treatments would be discussed with next of kin. If there is no time to do more to assess capacity, and severe distress impairs the ability to make a rational decision, treatment should be initiated to save her life even without consent. A court of law is likely to be more critical of fatal inactivity than well-intentioned care. However in most situations assessment of capacity is possible and all doctors should be conversant with the local Mental Capacity legislation.

In some countries even capacitous patients may be treated against their will using appropriate *mental health legislation* if they have a mental disorder and that disorder is posing a risk to their health, their own safety or the safety of others. For e.g. the MHA in England and Wales would enable this patient to be detained (not investigated or treated) on the medical ward using Section 5(2) for up to 72 hours but the application needs to be made by the doctor in charge of the patient's care and not by the psychiatrist. To enable investigations and/or treatment against her will an application for admission under Section 2 or 3 of MHA will be needed. Section 2 or 3 will need an application by an approved mental health professional (usually a social worker) based on recommendations made by two doctors (one is usually a psychiatrist and the other usually the patient's general practitioner though in this case may be the treating physician). Section 2 is mainly an assessment section though treatment may also be provided under the act. Section 3 is a treatment section and may not be appropriate in this case, as any psychiatric diagnosis – if she has one at all is still provisional. Treatment under Sections 2 or 3 of the MHA can be given for mental disorders, but not physical conditions unless they are causing the mental disorder.

Appropriate local legislation should be used to assess and treat her without her consent if she has the capacity to refuse treatment but is suspected of suffering from a mental disorder impairing her safety.

Key Points

- Appropriate capacity legislation should be used to investigate or treat patients against their will. If a patient has capacity it is unlawful to give the patient treatment against his or her wishes even if the decision seems unwise.
- Appropriate mental health legislation may be used to treat medical conditions directly causing a mental disorder, or if the medical symptoms are a manifestation of a mental disorder even when the patient has full capacity to refuse treatment.

CASE 37: DISINHIBITED AND BEHAVING ODDLY

History

A 50-year-old part-time gardener attends the general practitioner (GP) surgery with his girlfriend. He announces that he has no complaints but is attending at the behest of his girlfriend. She tearfully says that over the past year, he has been behaving 'very oddly' and in a socially embarrassing and tactless manner. He has openly flirted with other women in her presence, at times making lewd remarks about their breasts or legs. He has been sacked from two weekend jobs for behaving 'inappropriately' but he says that he likes women and sees no harm in 'trying his luck'. He seems oblivious to the pain his actions are causing his girlfriend. When she continues to sob, he turns to her and shouts at her angrily, accusing her of being 'silly'. He then breaks down in tears himself.

He is facing disciplinary action at work and has been off work for the past 3 weeks. He has little motivation to return to work. His energy levels are good. He is sleeping well though his appetite has decreased over the past 6 months and he has lost half a stone in weight. He has had intermittent headaches but otherwise there is no significant medical history. There is no history of any psychiatric illness. He smokes 20 cigarettes a day but does not abuse alcohol or any illicit drugs. He lives with his girlfriend in a council maisonette. He has debts worth £3000, but is not 'bothered' about it. Physical examination is unremarkable.

Mental state examination

He seems irritable and it is difficult to establish a rapport. His speech is coherent, relevant but slow. He displays psychomotor retardation. He does not have formal thought disorder or any other psychotic symptoms. His mood appears labile varying from low to mildly euphoric and irritable. He is orientated in time, place and person. His attention span and concentration are impaired as evidenced by serial sevens test. When asked to name words beginning with the letter 'F', he names six words in 1 minute (normal range 10–20 seconds) indicating impaired verbal fluency. He is unable to perform reciprocal tasks (tapping once when the examiner taps twice and tapping twice when the examiner taps once) or alternating tasks (alternately drawing triangles and rectangles).

Questions

- What is the likely diagnosis?
- What are the differential diagnoses?
- How would you manage this patient?

ANSWER 37

This man is presenting with sub-acute onset of socially disinhibited behaviour, lack of empathy, insensitivity, impaired judgement, poor motivation and lability of mood representing a significant change in his personality. Organic disorders should always be suspected in late-onset personality changes. Orbitofrontal lesions are characterized by disinhibition, mood lability and impulsivity while frontal convexity lesions show apathy, indifference and psychomotor slowing. In practice, a significant overlap is seen in frontal lobe dysfunction, as is the case in this man. Cognitive examination showing impaired concentration, impaired verbal fluency and impaired frontal system tasks such as reciprocal or alternate programmes further suggests frontal lobe pathology. A diagnosis of organic personality disorder is most likely. A range of causes of frontal lobe pathology must be considered including stroke, head trauma, cerebral tumors, epilepsy, Huntington disease, multiple sclerosis, endocrine disorders, neurosyphilis and acquired immune deficiency syndrome (AIDS). In this case, intermittent headaches and weight loss point in the direction of a cerebral tumour. Other psychiatric differentials of frontal lobe pathology or disinhibited behaviour need to be ruled out, such as

- Alzheimer's dementia involving global deterioration in cognition and behaviour rather than change mainly in personality.
- Pick disease, which is a frontotemporal dementia.
- Manic episode including elated/irritable mood, psychomotor agitation, flights of ideas, grandiosity and reduced sleep. There may be a previous history of mood episode.
- Mixed affective disorder is an intermix of manic and depressive symptoms in the same episode. Again, a previous history of mood episode and an episodic course point to this diagnosis.

In management the first step is to identify the underlying cause for which a further history, blood screen and brain scan (computed tomography [CT]/magnetic resonance imaging [MRI]) is essential. Comprehensive mental state examination may occasionally need to be supplemented by expert neuropsychological testing to differentiate medical from non-medical psychiatric pathology. If a neurological/medical cause is identified, referral to the relevant department is indicated. If psychiatric symptoms are predominant, as in this case, referral to and joint working with the liaison psychiatry team are useful. Treating the underlying cause (if treatable) is the key management strategy. Additionally symptomatic treatment may be indicated where symptoms are distressing or disabling. In this case, he is displaying lability of mood and agitation for which he can be prescribed an antipsychotic medication such as quetiapine. Antidepressants may be needed if depression seems to predominate in the clinical picture. His girlfriend is very worried and will benefit from a carer's assessment and subsequent support.

Key Points

- Late-onset personality change is often associated with frontal lobe dysfunction; careful cognitive testing is needed to establish this.
- Treating the underlying cause and symptomatic treatment is the key management strategies.

CASE 38: WHAT IS GOING ON IN THIS CONSULTATION?

History

A 50-year-old married woman presents with poorly controlled diabetes. The woman insists that she is putting all the advice given to her in place but that it is not helping her diabetes. She wonders whether it would be better managed if she saw you weekly. She also insists that she is not helped by seeing different members of the clinical team and that it would be better if she just saw you. You find yourself struggling to understand how the fairly straightforward dietary advice cannot be implemented by the woman as she clearly understands what is required. She seems very competent but insists that without your help she cannot manage. She is married but has recently had problems with her husband who has had considerable health problems of his own. She says that he does not understand her health problems and is preoccupied with his own difficulties. You get the impression she feels somewhat let down by him as she was by her father who left the family when she was only 8 years old and failed to maintain any regular contact. On one occasion she leaves a message with the reception that says: 'I need to see you urgently. You are the only one that understands.'

Her need to be seen and approved by you makes you uncomfortable, and you are struggling with how to manage this and move forward.

Mental state examination

She is well-dressed and although her hair is not tidy, she has used a lot of makeup. She makes good and sometimes intense eye contact. She presents as over-familiar, calling you by your first name. She begins the appointment by presenting you with a cake she has baked especially for you. When you hesitate to accept it, she urges you to take it as not doing so will be too much for her to cope with. There is no evidence of speech or mood disorder and she is not psychotic.

Questions

- What might be happening here?
- Why is it important to reflect on how you are feeling?

ANSWER 38

It may be helpful to reflect on this woman's needs in terms of relationships. Understanding the situation in terms of transference may be helpful. Transference is a phenomenon described in psychoanalysis, which is characterized by the unconscious redirection of feelings for one person to another. This transference projects feelings, emotions or motivations onto another person without realizing that much of it emanates from within the self (and past relationships).

Typically, the pattern projected onto the other person comes from a childhood relationship. This may be from an actual person, such as a parent, or an idealized figure or prototype. This transfers both power and expectation with both positive and negative outcomes. Exploring the situations and whom we place our transference on can identify our real motives and thoughts. What we read into other people reveals our secret prejudices and our unfulfilled wishes. Transference occurs on a regular basis but is particularly useful as a therapeutic tool to promote self-understanding.

Counter-transference is the response that is elicited in the recipient (therapist) by the other's (patient) unconscious transference communications. Transference also provides a good idea of what the patient might be expecting from you. In this case scenario, the fact that the patient wants to see you weekly may mean she depends on you in a way that she wishes she could depend on her partner. That may in the longer term be a problem because while she is investing in you, it may make it difficult for her to address the real issues of her relationship with her partner. However, it can be useful because it may help her understand that she is visiting you with relatively trivial complaints because she has unmet emotional needs.

Feelings are easier to identify if they are not congruent with the doctor's personality and expectation of his or her role. Doctors may struggle with transference since they may have a need themselves to feel needed. They may unwittingly encourage this and only realize the impact once a degree of dependency has been created. This may only emerge when several similar doctor–patient relationships have arisen. If they lack awareness they may react emotionally with irritation, rather than consider the role they might also have played in establishing this dynamic. Awareness of the transference–counter-transference relationship allows a more considered response. Being aware of the subconscious patient agenda may help the doctor recognize some of the patient's wishes and fears and address these openly and sensitively. It may also help explain certain behaviours from both the patient and doctor. Understanding this also means that the doctor is able to step back and avoid feeling overwhelmed by excessive patient demand as he or she has greater awareness of what might be happening.

Key Points

- Transference happens in most relationships.
- Not recognizing transference and counter-transference can have a negative impact on the doctor–patient relationship.

CASE 39: THINGS ARE GETTING WORSE

A 24-year-old engineering student attends the psychiatric follow-up clinic complaining of sudden jerky movement of his limbs over the past 3 weeks. He was diagnosed with depression 8 months ago and has been treated with fluoxetine 40 mg a day, without much benefit. Three months ago he started becoming more withdrawn and suspicious. He was referred to the Early Intervention in Psychosis Team who did not find any evidence of psychosis but suggested schizoid personality with depression. Risperidone 3 mg a day was added. He started developing mild dystonia; procyclidine 5 mg twice daily was commenced but the jerks progressively became worse. Stopping the risperidone and procyclidine made no difference. Presently, he also complains of funny sensations in his face and neck. His girlfriend feels that he is progressively becoming clumsy and losing balance, and is also quite forgetful. He lives with his girlfriend, does not abuse drugs or alcohol and has no previous psychiatric or medical history. His Mini Mental State Examination (MMSE) score is 20 out of 30, losing points on orientation, attention and memory.

Investigations

	Levels	*Reference range*
Haemoglobin	12.8 g/dL	11.7–15.7 g/dL
Mean corpuscular volume (MCV)	95 fL	80–99 fL
White cell count	7.8×10^9/L	$3.5–11.0 \times 10^9$/L
Platelets	220×10^9/L	$150–440 \times 10^9$/L
Erythrocyte sedimentation rate (ESR)	8 mm/h	<10 mm/h
Sodium	140 mmol/L	135–145 mmol/L
Potassium	4.2 mmol/L	3.5–5 mmol/L
Urea	5 mmol/L	2.5–6.7 mmol/L
Creatinine	98 μmol/L	70–120 μmol/L
Glucose	4.8 mmol/L	4.0–6.0 mmol/L
Lumbar puncture Leucocytes	4/mL	<5/mL
Cerebrospinal fluid (CSF) proteins	0.3 g/L	<0.4 g/L
CSF glucose plasma glucose value	4.4 mmol/L	>70%

Note: Computed tomography (CT) of the brain: normal. Electroencephalogram (EEG): diffuse slowing with spikes and sharp waves.

Questions

- What is the likely diagnosis?
- How will you manage this patient?

ANSWER 39

This young man has presented with depression but has gone on to develop myoclonic jerks, unsteady gait and cognitive deterioration. Family history should be taken for Huntington disease. An absent trauma history and no CT scan findings make Wilson's disease, multiple sclerosis, trauma or vascular causes unlikely. Normal blood chemistry and normal CSF should raise suspicion of a rare cause of dementia. Drug side effects may cause some symptoms but not to this extent. This makes variant Creutzfeldt–Jakob disease (vCJD) a possibility. vCJD is one of four human spongiform encephalopathies (so called on account of the spongy appearance of brain tissue on autopsy). These are prion diseases, so called as the infective agent prion and a form of its protein called PrP (prion protein) have been implicated in causation. The other types include sporadic CJD (most common), genetic CJD and iatrogenic CJD (caused by treatment with cadaveric-derived human growth hormone or the use of human dura mater graft in surgery or blood transfusion from infected patients or the use of infected instruments in surgery). vCJD differs from sporadic CJD in that there is younger age of onset, longer course and psychiatric presentation as is the case in this patient.

Brain biopsy is diagnostic but rarely feasible. Diagnosis is suspected in cases of negative findings for other causes of young-onset dementia. Sporadic CJD shows characteristic 'periodic complexes' on EEG. These are generalized bi- or triphasic periodic sharp wave complexes occurring at a frequency of 1–2 per second. However, this finding is not seen in vCJD. Diagnosis depends on identification of bilateral symmetrical hyperintensity in the pulvinar (posterior) nuclei of the thalamus. The 'pulvinar sign' on magnetic resonance imaging (MRI) brain scan is seen in 90% of cases (see Figure 39.1). Another supportive diagnostic test is tonsil biopsy, which reveals the offending prion protein. Also suggestive is the presence of a particular protein called 14-3-3 in CSF.

The National CJD Surveillance Unit (in the United Kingdom) or a similar public health body should be notified once the disease is suspected as the patient is 'at risk' for public health purposes. He should be advised that he would not be able to carry out blood or organ donation.

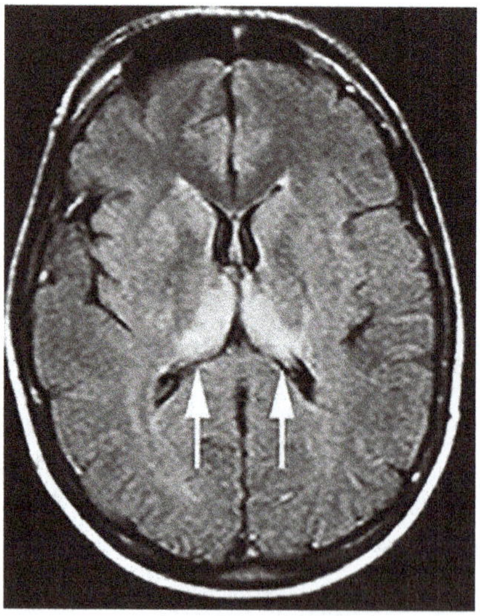

Figure 39.1 The pulvinar sign – symmetrical hyperintensity in the posterior nuclei of the thalamus.

There is no specific treatment for CJD although drugs such as quinacrine and pentosan polysulphate have been used on an individual basis. Psychiatric syndromes or symptoms may need appropriate treatment. This includes antipsychotic medication for agitation or psychotic symptoms, antidepressants for low mood and benzodiazepines for movement disorder and anxiety. Physiotherapists and speech therapists can help with dysphagia, dysarthria and dyspraxia. Referral to a support network facilitates provision of support to patients and carers. This is a neurodegenerative disorder and as the disease progresses, functional ability reduces progressively and patients ultimately need full-time nursing care. Social services should therefore be involved at an early stage.

Key Points

- CJD, especially vCJD, often presents with psychiatric symptoms.
- CT scan is normal; however, MRI reveals the characteristic pulvinar sign.

CASE 40: DIARRHOEA AND VOMITING AFTER IRREGULAR EATING

History

A 21-year-old woman presents in the emergency department with acute abdominal pain and vomiting and diarrhoea. The pain is cramping in nature. The diarrhoea and vomiting have been present for 2 days without any abatement. Prior to this her eating has been very variable. Sometimes she goes for the whole day without eating as she does not like eating in public. Occasionally she gets ravenous and eats large quantities of junk food (e.g. whole packets of biscuits and cakes). She then tends to feel guilty and says that the guilt makes her feel sick. She does not like how she looks as she feels she is much bigger than her peers and she cannot wear current fashions as well as they can. She has not been on holiday and has not been unwell, although is gradually feeling weaker. She denies being on any prescribed medication but says she had been taking a herbal remedy to clear her bowels as part of a detoxification programme. Recently she says she is not depressed, can enjoy herself and has no thoughts of self-harm. She has not used any illicit drugs, does not smoke and only occasionally consumes alcohol. There is no other previous history of note.

Physical examination

The woman looks dehydrated. She has no fever. Her pulse is 84 beats per minute and her blood pressure is 130/70 mm Hg. Her body mass index (BMI) is 24.9 (height 152 cm, weight 58 kg). She has calluses on her knuckles (which she states she got having hit her hand on a wall). Her teeth are discoloured and in poor condition.

Her abdomen is not tender, and rectal examination shows that she is constipated.

Investigations

	Levels	*Reference range*
Haemoglobin	12.8 g/dL	11.7–15.7 g/dL
White cell count	8.8 × 10^9/L	3.5–11.0 × 10^9/L
Platelets	280 × 10^9/L	150–440 × 10^9/L
Sodium	139 mmol/L	135–145 mmol/L
Potassium	3.1 mmol/L	3.5–5.0 mmol/L
Urea	4.4 mmol/L	2.5–6.7 mmol/L
Glucose	5.3 mmol/L	4.0–6.0 mmol/L
Creatinine	75 µmol/L	70–120 µmol/L
Alkaline phosphatase	88 IU/L	30–300 IU/L
Alanine aminotransferase	12 IU/L	5–35 IU/L
Gamma-glutamyl transpeptidase	32 IU/L	11–51 IU/L

Questions

- What is the differential diagnosis?
- What are the treatment options?

ANSWER 40

When considering the gastrointestinal presentation, many things are ruled out by history, examination and investigations. These include gastrointestinal problems (especially upper gastrointestinal tract) such as infection or repeated vomiting as a result of physical disorders (e.g. right ventricular failure). Prolonged starvation does not fit with the BMI. Anxiety or depression should be monitored but given her history bulimia is the most likely diagnosis. The hypokalaemia and signs on the knuckles and teeth are likely caused by repeated self-induced vomiting. The purging type is the most likely as she has been making herself sick and she may also have been using diuretics to control her weight.

Hypokalaemia can be caused by the sudden uptake of potassium ions from the bloodstream by muscle or other organs or by an overall depletion of the body's potassium. The most common cause of hypokalaemia is diuretics. Other common causes of hypokalaemia are excessive diarrhoea, enema abuse or vomiting. It can also occur in medical conditions such as diabetes (ketoacidosis), adrenal tumours, hyperaldosteronism and renal artery stenosis, although these can be ruled out by history and investigation. Up to 20% of people complaining of chronic diarrhoea practise laxative abuse. Laxative abuse is often part of eating disorders, such as anorexia nervosa or bulimia nervosa. Hypokalaemia in eating disorders may be life-threatening with symptoms ranging from lethargy and cloudy thinking to cardiac arrhythmias and death.

The acute management will be to medically stabilize this woman. She will need to be carefully monitored while she is assessed and treated. Treatment of the hypokalaemia involves addressing the cause, in this case psychoeducation about the risk this woman is putting herself in. High-potassium food such as oranges and bananas can be used for mild hypokalaemia (not below 3 mmol/L) with oral potassium supplementation if necessary. If her potassium levels were below 2.5 mmol/L, intravenous potassium should be given. The speed of administration should be slow to avoid rapid changes in potassium levels, which can trigger adverse events such as arrhythmias. Regardless she will need referral for the support and management of her bulimia nervosa.

In bulimia there is often a lack of control over eating, sometimes to the point of physical discomfort. Eating patterns are often not healthy and may be covert. There may be signs of purging such as going to the bathroom after meals to vomit and overt or covert use of laxatives or diuretics. These all need to be addressed.

! Medical complications and adverse effects of bulimia

- Weight gain
- Abdominal pain, bloating
- Chronic sore throat, hoarseness
- Tooth decay and mouth sores
- Broken blood vessels in the eyes
- Swollen cheeks and salivary glands
- Acid reflux or ulcers
- Weakness and dizziness
- Amenorrhoea

The most usual treatment is cognitive behaviour therapy with counselling and support, but there are several other bulimia treatments that are effective. Interpersonal psychotherapy helps people with bulimia solve relationship issues and interpersonal problems that are contributing to their eating disorder. Interpersonal psychotherapy may also help depression and low self-esteem which are common with bulimia. Group therapy is helpful in bulimia treatment involving education about the eating disorder and strategies for overcoming it. Self-help and support groups are also of benefit. If there is co-morbid depression, consider using selective serotonin reuptake inhibitors (SSRIs).

Key Points

- Bulimia is often well hidden and may present through medical complications.
- There is often co-morbidity especially with depression, substance misuse and emotionally unstable personality disorder.

CASE 41: FEVER AND CONFUSION

History

A 24-year-old postgraduate student has been admitted to the inpatient psychiatric unit for the past 4 days following a relapse of schizophrenia. Over the last 2 days he has been getting increasingly agitated and paranoid, accusing the nursing staff and other patients of poisoning him. He has refused food and drink and has attacked a member of staff. His first episode, 3 years ago, had resolved successfully with olanzapine (atypical antipsychotic medication). However, he had stopped taking this medication 3 weeks prior to admission. On admission, he was prescribed oral quetiapine 300 mg at night with haloperidol orally 5 mg three times daily in case of agitation along with lorazepam orally or intramuscularly (IM) 1–2 mg up to four times daily as required. He refused to take oral olanzapine and was administered haloperidol 5 mg three times daily IM with lorazepam 1 mg twice daily and 2 mg at nighttime IM over the last 2 days. Despite this, his agitation has been increasing and his speech has become more incoherent and bizarre. He was also prescribed procyclidine 5 mg twice daily after the duty doctor assessed him 2 days ago.

Mental state examination

He was assessed by the duty trainee doctor and was found to have irrelevant and incoherent speech with formal thought disorder. His eye contact was fleeting. He was disorientated and had no insight. He has a number of clear paranoid delusions and is responding to auditory hallucinations but is unable to describe them. He has little insight into his illness.

Physical examination

He was found to have tachycardia (120 beats per minute) and raised blood pressure (160/104 mm Hg). Core body temperature was 39°C. Central nervous system (CNS) examination revealed extrapyramidal muscle rigidity assumed to be secondary to antipsychotic medication, with a generalized tremor that was attributed to agitation and anxiety. Further systemic examination did not reveal any other abnormality.

Investigations

	Levels	*Reference range*
Haemoglobin	12.2 g/dL	11.7–15.7 g/dL
White blood cell count	17.2×10^9/L	$3.5–11.0 \times 10^9$/L
Sodium	137 mmol/L	135–145 mmol/L
Potassium	4.6 mmol/L	3.5–5.0 mmol/L
Thyroid-stimulating hormone	3.5 mU/L	0.3–6.0 mU/L
Urea	6.0 mmol/L	2.5–6.7 mmol/L
Creatinine	84 µmol/L	70–120 µmol/L
Alkaline phosphatase	84 IU/L	30–300 IU/L
Alkaline aminotransferase	30 IU/L	5–35 IU/L
Creatine phosphokinase	10,000 IU/L	30–200 IU/L

Questions

- What is the differential diagnosis?
- How will you manage this patient?
- How will you manage his schizophrenia in the future?

ANSWER 41

This man has hyperpyrexia, autonomic dysfunction (tachycardia, sweating, raised blood pressure, tremors), muscle rigidity and mental confusion. This tetrad of symptoms is highly suggestive of an idiosyncratic reaction to antipsychotic medication known as neuroleptic malignant syndrome (NMS). The central pathology is severe dopaminergic blockade leading to extreme muscle rigidity, which may cause rhabdomyolysis (muscle tissue breakdown) and acute renal failure. Early recognition of this medical emergency is vital as it can be fatal in up to 20% of cases.

! Higher risk of NMS

- The use of typical antipsychotics (though atypicals are not completely safe).
- Rapid upward titrations in dose.
- Withdrawal of anticholinergic medication.
- Depot preparations.
- Dehydration.
- High ambient temperature.
- Past episode of NMS.
- Males have twice the risk of females.

Differential diagnoses include infections such as meningitis, encephalitis, and septicaemia with or without concurrent extrapyramidal rigidity. Neuroendocrine possibilities include thyrotoxicosis and phaeochromocytoma. It could be drug induced with toxicity from illicit drugs (e.g. cocaine and amphetamines) or prescription drugs (e.g. salicylates and anticholinergic medication). Heat stroke or malignant hyperthermia should be considered. Also exclude neuropsychiatric presentations such as status epilepticus and catatonia (secondary to mood disorder or schizophrenia). Diagnosis is facilitated by a high index of clinical suspicion. Monitoring all patients on antipsychotic medication for extrapyramidal side effects is vital. The presence of any other feature such as fever, confusion or autonomic dysfunction should lead to a detailed physical examination and investigations to rule out the above differentials. Useful investigations include the following (findings in NMS in parentheses): full blood count (leucocytosis), urea and electrolytes (raised in renal failure), liver function tests (raised serum transaminases), creatinine kinase (raised in renal failure) and urine drug screen to rule out drug intoxication.

Management

This is a medical emergency and will require urgent transfer to a medical unit. Maintaining ABC (airway, breathing and circulation) is vital. The antipsychotic medication should be discontinued immediately. Maintain hydration with intravenous fluids and maintain temperature with antipyretics and cooling devices. Dialysis is necessary in renal failure. There is some evidence to show the utility of generalized muscle relaxants such as dantrolene as well as for the use of dopaminergic medications such as amantadine.

Future psychiatric treatment will involve treating schizophrenia with antipsychotic medications, which carry a high risk of NMS. Treatment should therefore be commenced in an inpatient setting only 2 weeks after successful resolution of current NMS. Long-acting or depot preparations should be avoided. Use low-dose atypical antipsychotic medication and titrate the dose upwards slowly.

Key Points

- Hyperpyrexia, autonomic dysfunction, muscle rigidity and mental confusion with antipsychotic exposure suggest a diagnosis of NMS.
- Maintaining ABC and symptomatic treatment in the medical setting are helpful.
- Restart antipsychotic medication under close supervision as a psychiatry inpatient.

CASE 42: 'ALIEN IMPULSES' AND RISK TO OTHERS

History

A 30-year-old shop assistant presents to the emergency department requesting that they remove the microchip from her brain. She says that this chip was implanted into her brain some weeks ago in order that aliens could control her mind.

She has previously been diagnosed with paranoid schizophrenia and has had a number of previous admissions to psychiatric hospitals, the majority of which have been involuntary admissions. She has previously been treated with a number of different types of antipsychotic medications, and this is currently olanzapine 20 mg once daily. Her last admission to hospital was 6 months ago and since this time she has often missed her medication. She has no past medical history of note.

There is no family history of mental illness. She is currently living with her parents who are supportive of her. From the ages of 18 to 28 she smoked high-potency cannabis ('skunk') on an almost daily basis, but following advice and support from her community mental health team she has successfully cut down her use of cannabis to approximately once every month. She has no other history of alcohol or illicit substance abuse. Although she has no previous convictions she has previously assaulted her parents and ward nursing staff when psychotic.

Mental state examination

She presents as unkempt and is surprised that she is being asked about her previous psychiatric history rather than being referred to a neurosurgeon for removal of the microchip. Despite this it is possible to establish a good rapport. At several points during the interview she stops speaking in mid-sentence and stares intently into one of the corners of the room and begins whispering to herself.

She believes that a microchip has been implanted into her brain and that aliens are using this to 'put things into my mind'. She describes how the aliens put impulses into her mind which she feels compelled to act upon. For 2 days the 'alien impulses' have concentrated on killing her mother and she is concerned that she may act upon these. She denies any hallucinations but during the interview appears to be responding to unseen auditory stimuli. She has little insight and does not accept that a relapse of her mental illness could be responsible for her current difficulties. There is no abnormality upon physical examination.

Questions

- What psychopathological term could be used to describe her belief that aliens are putting impulses into her brain which she must act on?
- How would you assess the risk that this patient may pose to others?

ANSWER 42

Her belief that impulses are being put into her brain and are no longer under her control is an example of passivity. The term *passivity* is used when the patient has the delusion that some aspect that is normally under his or her own control is instead controlled by an external agency. Examples of passivity phenomena are made impulses, made feelings and somatic passivity (a delusion that part of the body is under external control). Thought passivity refers to the belief that thoughts are inserted, removed or blocked.

There are indications from this patient's presentation and history that she may pose a risk to others and in particular her mother. She is experiencing passivity phenomena that include the made impulse to kill her mother. In addition to this she has a history of assaults upon others (including her parents) when unwell. Her risk to others is also increased by her lack of insight, poor compliance and history of cannabis abuse.

A comprehensive risk assessment is essential in this case. In order to do this it is important to obtain relevant information from as many sources as possible. This could include a more detailed history and mental state examination from the patient, discussion with an informant (her parents would be especially helpful in this case) and previous psychiatric and medical records and information from any professionals recently involved in her care (such as community psychiatric nurse, social worker or general practitioner). This information should then be used to evaluate the presence/absence of relevant risk factors.

! Examples of relevant risk-increasing factors

- History of previous violence
- Substance abuse
- Psychotic illness
- Personality disorder
- Anger
- Lack of social support
- Relationship or employment problems
- Evidence of early maladjustment
- Non-compliance with treatment
- Use of/access to weapons
- Negative attitudes and violent fantasies
- Impulsivity
- Lack of insight

Other areas of risk that should be explored include risk of harm to self or suicide, risk of exploitation and risk of neglect. A summary judgement of risk should then be made. This should include what the risk is, who is at risk and the likelihood of this harm occurring. From this should follow an appropriate risk management plan. In this case it would be appropriate to consider admitting the patient to hospital. Given the risk here, if this offer is declined consider involuntary admission using appropriate legislation, e.g. the Mental Health Act (1983) in England.

Key Points

- Passivity phenomena involve the patient believing that some aspect of his or her body or mind is under the control of an external agency.
- Comprehensive risk assessment should involve information from several sources and will lead on to appropriate risk management and the provision of appropriate clinical care.

CASE 43: FEELS LIKE THE ROOM IS CHANGING SHAPE

History

A 19-year-old woman comes to clinic and describes that she is worried by experiences where the usual sounds in the room begin to fluctuate in intensity, almost like they are coming from a radio with the sound being altered. There is no radio present. This lasts for about 10 minutes and then she gets a severe throbbing headache. More commonly, on other occasions she has had the strange experience that her body is changing shape and becoming smaller and that she is farther away from the walls, even though she knows that the room has not actually changed shape. Sometimes this comes with a sensation that time is rushing past. Again she subsequently has a powerful headache that throbs and is usually unilateral. She reports no recent stressful life events and has worked at a supermarket checkout for 15 months. She has a healthy group of friends.

There is no history of epilepsy or drug abuse, although she drinks up to 20 units of alcohol a week, usually over two nights at the weekend. The episodes do not occur in this context. There is no family history of epilepsy but a strong family history of migraine. Her mother has classical migraine with throbbing headaches, photophobia and vomiting. Her father reports having visual shimmering for 20–30 minutes about five times a year, but has no headaches associated with this.

Mental state examination

The 19-year-old woman is well dressed, clean and wears some light makeup. She makes normal eye contact and has healthy behaviour with no agitation or psychomotor retardation. Her mood is euthymic both subjectively and objectively. She would like to know what the symptoms mean. She is worried that she might be going mad. Other than the symptoms that she has described there is no evidence of any unusual or strange psychopathology.

A full neurological examination is normal.

Investigations

	Levels	*Reference range*
Haemoglobin	13.9 g/dL	11.7–15.7 g/dL
Mean corpuscular volume (MCV)	85 fL	80–99 fL
White cell count	4.6×10^9/L	$3.5–11.0 \times 10^9$/L
Platelets	302×10^9/L	$150–440 \times 10^9$/L
Glucose	5.3 mmol/L	4.0–6.0 mmol/L
Urine drug screen	Negative	

Note: Electroencephalogram: normal; computed tomography scan of the head: normal.

Questions

- Are her experiences illusions or hallucinations?
- What is the differential diagnosis?
- What is the most likely diagnosis?

ANSWER 43

The distortions of the ambient sounds are illusions. They are distortions of real perceptions. They would only be hallucinations if they occurred in the absence of external stimuli and were perceived as a true perception in external space (i.e. not a thought or an imagined sound). Similarly macropsia describes the sensation that objects are larger (and the person smaller in relation) than normal. Micropsia is the reverse.

! Hallucinations and illusions

- *Hallucination*: a sensory perception in the absence of an external stimulus that is experienced as a real perception
- *Illusion*: a mistaken or false interpretation of a real sensory experience that usually comes about when a person's imagined or expected perceptions merge with real perception

The differential diagnoses would include complex partial epilepsy, psychoactive drug use (e.g. cannabis or magic mushrooms), migraine, early psychosis, severe sleep deprivation, severe stress, space-occupying lesion or feigned illness.

In this example, there is no history of drug misuse, and the urine screen is negative. There is no additional psychopathology indicative of psychosis, although this should be monitored at future visits. Further tests were discussed but mutually agreed not to be necessary.

The general practitioner referred the patient to a neurologist who diagnosed migraine using the term 'Alice in Wonderland syndrome'. This was coined by Todd in 1955, because of the various instances of metamorphopsia, micropsia and macropsia described in the tale where Alice perceived herself to be smaller, changing shape and objects around her to be changing in size. In Chapter 5 of Lewis Carroll's book, Alice encounters a caterpillar sitting on a mushroom, smoking 'Hookah'. This is of note given that the toadstool *Amanita muscaria* has hallucinogenic properties. Carroll wrote of his own migrainous headaches in later life. In fact while migrainous auras are commonly known to include scotomata, or transient speech or power loss, it should be remembered that the spreading depression that is associated with aura can happen anywhere in the brain, and therefore can create a range of other symptoms (that are either less common or less commonly reported).

The treatment for migraine involves analgesics such as paracetamol and non-steroidal anti-inflammatory drugs. Antiemetics are useful if nausea is a key part. Serotonin agonists that cause cerebral vasoconstriction can be helpful for some people. Prophylaxis such as beta-blockers, tricyclics and the anticonvulsant topiramate can be effective, although there is a high rate of placebo response found in comparative studies.

In Alice in Wonderland syndrome knowing the diagnosis is a great help to patients as it reassures them that they do not have a severe mental illness and that they do not have epilepsy. Prevention may be helped by recognizing particular triggers such as tiredness or diet, and making lifestyle changes accordingly. Rarely, other triggers have been reported such as physical exercise or bright lights.

Key Point

- Migraine aura can affect different parts of the brain other than visual centres. This can produce a range of rare but migraine-related symptoms.

CASE 44: UNABLE TO OPEN MY FISTS

History

A 19-year-old woman presents to her general practitioner (GP) saying that she is unable to open her fists. She says that 3 days ago she woke up and found it to be like this. She says she also started to see in black and white for a few hours and could see no colours. She explains that she has been otherwise healthy recently. Her records indicate that she has presented regularly to the GP in the past. The last five presentations have been for an ear infection, pains on the soles of both feet, shoulder pain, restless legs at night and neck pain. She has a cousin with cerebral palsy and her grandfather had a stroke 1 year ago and is now in a wheelchair. Further questioning reveals no other neurological symptoms. She did not do well in General Certificate of Secondary Education examinations and required extra help at school in the past for learning. She started work at a supermarket and was recently promoted to the check-out. She says that she does not like this, and prefers being on shelf-stacking duties. Her father is known to the practice as someone who has significant problems with alcohol dependence syndrome. Systematic enquiry for depression is unremarkable. She does describe some anxiety about work but has great difficulty articulating it.

Physical and mental state examination

The fists are tightly closed and on gentle examination it is not possible to open the fingers. There is clear resistance to movement. The woman does not appear to be unduly concerned. A neurological examination reveals no other abnormalities. Tone in all other limbs and muscle groups appears normal. Her reflexes are all normal. There are no visual field defects. There is no evidence of status epilepticus. She chats and answers questions asked of her.

On mental state examination she makes good eye contact and smiles readily. She sits with her fists clenched as if holding ski poles with the thumbs slightly rotated into the midline. There is no agitation, restlessness or retardation of movements. She does not fidget and there is no evidence of tics or other movement problems. She describes no low mood and appears euthymic. There is no evidence of thought passivity, hallucinations or delusions. When asked what she thinks is wrong she says: 'I am paralysed in my hands'.

Questions

- How would her symptoms be explained neurologically?
- What is the most likely diagnosis?
- What are the elements of good management?

ANSWER 44

There are no good explanations for her symptoms neurologically. A motor lesion in the brain would cause a unilateral loss of control and this would usually be a flaccid loss of power, with contractures only developing over time with lack of movement. The bilateral loss of colour vision (acquired achromatopsia) is neurologically explainable by bilateral lesions in the visual cortex, and is exceptionally rare. It is usually accompanied by visual field defects and other signs.

The most likely diagnosis is a conversion disorder resulting in loss of power. It is possible that this occurs against a backdrop of somatization disorder, where a range of symptoms occur across time. This is thought to represent physical expression of psychological distress. It is also possible that this is feigned and that the symptom provides significant gain for the person (either allowing her to avoid a predicament or a stressful circumstance, or giving financial reward or sick leave). Please also check other cases involving aspects of somatization (e.g. 18, 44, 60 and 81).

Conversion disorder often occurs with co-morbid anxiety and/or depression, and even though you have not been able to identify this thus far, it is worth keeping an open mind and exploring this further. Some people will have 'belle indifference', meaning that they would be expected to be much more distressed about their symptoms than they appear to be, which may be the case here.

Joint management between a neurologist and a liaison psychiatrist or clinical psychologist would be the most common strategy. The neurologist can get a range of necessary examinations out of the way early. These allow the clinical team to move on and be confident in their diagnosis, which promotes the most effective management. In situations like this it is possible that relatively little investigation is necessary, with hefty reassurance and explanation to the woman concerned.

Most importantly take the symptom seriously. Positive attributions about recovery are fostered by strategies that are perceived as recovery inducing. For example, physiotherapy should be used and allied with strong 'seeding' of ideas about recovery. There should be careful exploration of any factors that may be contributing to the maintenance of the symptoms. Possible areas to explore would include relationships at home and working practices. Confrontation strategies do not seem to work very well and may lead to disengagement from services or additional symptomatology. Positive reinforcement of healthy functioning needs to be built into the programme. Therapy that allows the young woman to begin to understand links between stress/emotions and physical symptoms is helpful. This would include examples about stress headaches, high blood pressure, nail-biting, palpitations and peptic ulcers. This allows a discussion about very real physical symptoms being related to stress and psychological factors. This can then move on to discussions about stressors in her life. These might be as simple as moving onto the checkouts and not being able to say no, although they may be more complex. Family mechanisms may be important if dysfunction (e.g. in the context of an alcohol-dependent father) has altered relationships, communication or developmental learning of adaptive coping strategies. Medication is not helpful unless you have identified a clear need (e.g. clinical depression). Making sure that the team members work together with a common plan is important.

Key Points

- Conversion disorder can produce a range of symptoms and is different from feigned symptomatology in that psychological distress elicits physical symptoms without conscious intent.
- Management is multi-faceted.
- Medication is not usually useful unless there is a clear co-morbid condition such as depression.

CASE 45: INTENSE FATIGUE

History

A 23-year-old woman comes to see you with intense fatigue. She says it has been going on for 9 months, and started after a viral infection that she caught while on a visit to relatives. At the time she had a fever, sore throat, aching muscles and felt drained. While she initially seemed to recover and went back to work in an advertising agency, she has only been able to return to work part time for 2 weeks, and has been off continuously now for 7 months. She describes unrefreshing and disturbed sleep. She also describes feeling tired most of the time, generalized aches and feeling exhausted after even slight exercise. Her appetite is good and systemic enquiry reveals no other symptomatology.

Mental state examination

She makes good eye-to-eye contact. Her hair is tied up and does not look as though it has been washed for some time. She appears slightly on edge but answers all your questions openly. Her speech is normal in flow and content and she has no pressure of speech. She describes feeling fed up with being ill and low in mood. There is no suicidal ideation or intent. There is no thought passivity or any hallucinations either to observe or in the history. She also has no delusions. She does have a belief in poltergeists and wonders if there might be one in the house at the moment, because she has found things left out in the kitchen when she thought she had put them away.

Investigations

	Levels	*Reference range*
Haemoglobin	11.9 g/dL	11.7–15.7 g/dL
Mean corpuscular volume (MCV)	94 fL	80–99 fL
White cell count	5.2×10^9/L	$3.5–11.0 \times 10^9$/L
Platelets	292×10^9/L	$150–440 \times 10^9$/L
Thyroid-stimulating hormone	3.2 mU/L	0.3–6.0 mU/L
Free thyroxine	14.1 pmol/L	9.0–22.0 pmol/L
Glucose	4.7 mmol/L	4.0–6.0 mmol/L
Sodium	140 mmol/L	135–145 mmol/L
Potassium	3.9 mmol/L	3.5–5.0 mmol/L
Bicarbonate	26 mmol/L	24–30 mmol/L
Urea	4.9 mmol/L	2.5–6.7 mmol/L
Creatinine	76 μmol/L	70–120 μmol/L

Questions

- What possible diagnoses go through your mind?
- What further information would you need?

ANSWER 45

It is important to think broadly and remember that fatigue can be a component of a range of illnesses and social factors. Although the temptation is to think of a divide between physical and mental illnesses, very often physical illnesses have significant psychological consequences and if neurological, an effect on both physical and mental functioning. Similarly, mental health problems can lead to physical symptoms. Illnesses that should go through your mind include anaemia, diabetes, hypothyroidism and renal failure, but these have been excluded by investigations. Cardiac problems (including bradycardia and heart failure) need to be excluded by further history and an electrocardiogram. Cancer and infectious diseases may also need to be carefully excluded by systemic enquiry with any follow-up investigations as necessary. Other medical causes such as endocrine disorders, autoimmune disorders (such as myasthenia gravis) and cirrhosis or liver failure can be excluded by history, examination and investigation. Coeliac disease is unlikely since there is no anaemia. Other causes of malabsorption or malnutrition (e.g. an eating disorder) should also be excluded.

Clues to the most likely diagnosis lie in the history and include depression, infectious diseases or chronic fatigue syndrome. Chronic fatigue syndrome is sometimes called CFS/ME and refers to the same process (myalgic encephalopathy being a more popular but pathologically inaccurate term). Some believe it may be a heterogenous group and this is still being researched.

! Oxford criteria for CFS

- Severe disabling fatigue of at least 6 months' duration.
- Affects both physical and mental functioning.
- Present for more than 50% of the time.
- Myalgia, sleep and mood disturbances are sometimes present.
- Exclusion criteria include physical illnesses that cause fatigue, serious mental illness such as depression (low mood is not an exclusion criteria), dementia, psychosis or eating disorder.

Treatments on offer include pacing of energy usage, cognitive behaviour therapy, graded exercise and symptomatic medication. Different treatments are appropriate for different people. Various places have CFS teams that include a range of disciplines including physiotherapists, community nurses, occupational therapists, psychologists and psychiatrists who work together around agreed treatment protocols. Randomised controlled trials of medication (e.g. with antidepressants or immunoglobulins) either show no statistical differences or give equivocal results and have been difficult to replicate. Research shows that attributions about the illness appear in research to have an impact on outcomes. The most important factor appears to be a positive and empowering approach to treatment, with a good relationship between sufferer and clinician. It is important to avoid therapeutic nihilism and to collaboratively problem solve around therapeutic challenges.

Key Points

- There are no diagnostic tests for CFS.
- It is important to exclude other causes of fatigue.
- For diagnosis in children the Oxford criteria are used, but with 3 months as the minimum duration to ensure early diagnosis and treatment.

CASE 46: HALLUCINATIONS IN SOMEONE WITH EPILEPSY

History

You see a 27-year-old man who has epilepsy. He has a history of complex partial seizures. He has simple auditory hallucinations during the aura, but also psychotic symptoms between seizures. Prior to being on antipsychotic medication, after the seizures he would typically have a day when he felt well, and then would become unwell with auditory hallucinations, persecutory delusions, low mood and irritability. This would last for a few days. In the past he has also reported seeing fleeting images of people laughing at him.

Three years ago haloperidol was added to the antiepileptic medication phenytoin. His medication has kept him reasonably well. He is troubled with extrapyramidal side effects and has come to see you about this.

Questions

- What do you want to know to make a decision about his medication?
- What options do you have?

ANSWER 46

Psychosis and epilepsy

Epilepsy can be associated with psychosis particularly if the temporal lobes are affected. The psychosis can be

- Ictal (occurring during the seizure)
- Post-ictal (occurring after the seizure)
- Inter-ictal (persistent and not temporally related to seizures)

It is important to work with the patient and key carers to accurately record number, type, frequency and duration of seizures. This information should be recorded in a seizure diary. The precise nature of the psychotic symptoms and their temporal relationship with seizures should be recorded. It would be worth involving a community nurse in this work. It is also important to consider the patient's capacity and ability to consent to assessment and proposed treatment. You also need to know what extrapyramidal side-effects he is having.

It would be useful to ask for an electroencephalogram (EEG) and seek a neurology opinion on improving seizure control. Change of anticonvulsant medication may improve psychotic symptoms and it may be possible to withdraw or reduce haloperidol as a result. If an alternative anti-psychotic is considered, the practitioner should be aware of its effect on seizure threshold.

Unusual experiences in temporal lobe epilepsy

During the aura (seconds to minutes) the following may occur:

- Illusions or visual distortions.
- Hallucinations can be auditory, gustatory, olfactory or musical.
- Depersonalization or derealization or autoscopy (sensation of seeing one's own body).
- Strong emergence of memories.
- Déjà vu or amnesia.
- Strong emotions (e.g. anxiety, joy etc.) – some report powerful 'spiritual' experiences.

Complex partial seizures may include

- Impaired consciousness
- Repetitive movements and/or automatisms
- Lip smacking, mouth movements such as chewing and motionless staring
- Continuing with activities but without full awareness (fugue states)

There is sometimes generalization to tonic clonic seizures. There is usually post-ictal confusion and sleepiness.

Extrapyramidal and other side effects (see Case 96) can be unpleasant or distressing and may put patients off treatment that in other ways is working well for them. They may rarely be life threatening, especially if the dystonia affects muscles related to breathing (e.g. the larynx). Rarely, withdrawal dyskinesia may occur when medication is stopped.

Options for dealing with extrapyramidal side effects include reducing the dose, using more recently developed antipsychotic medication. In some instances a trial without neuroleptics is appropriate, especially if there has been good seizure control in the absence of psychotic experiences.

Key Points

- Psychotic symptoms may occur in relation to epilepsy.
- Accurately record seizures and improve seizure control.
- It is important to watch for extrapyramidal side effects in those taking antipsychotic medication.

CASE 47: I'M IMPOTENT

History

A 30-year-old man comes to see you in the general practitioner surgery. He is embarrassed and explains that he was married last year and is having problems with his sex life. In particular he mentions that since he was married he has had problems maintaining an erection when he is with his wife. He says that when he has been able to get an erection he often has a premature ejaculation. His wife has not been able to achieve orgasm. She has been very understanding and says that she does not mind, but he is concerned that there is something very wrong with him. He says that their relationship is good and he is very much in love with his wife. He has not told her that he is seeking advice. On further questioning he indicates that before he married he was a virgin, but that he did masturbate regularly and had sustained erections. He still occasionally masturbates in private and can sustain an erection for at least 5 minutes. His erections are normal and not painful. Brief systemic enquiry is normal. He has no polydipsia, polyuria, frequency, other urological symptoms or cardiovascular symptoms. He is an amateur football player who plays regularly and has not had any difficulties recently with fitness. He drinks socially at weekends only and is a non-smoker. He can still enjoy himself with his friends and his wife and denies any low mood. His work as owner of a small plumbing firm is going well.

Physical examination

He is clearly anxious and embarrassed. When you put him at his ease by explaining that the consultation is confidential and that this is a common problem with one in ten men experiencing it at some time, he becomes more relaxed. There is no evidence of any serious mental illness.

He has a pulse of 88 beats per minute and a blood pressure of 125/75 mm Hg. His heart sounds are normal. He is fit and appears healthy. His body mass index is 22. There are no penile, testicular or scrotal abnormalities, and he has normal muscle and hair distribution. The pulses in his legs and feet are normal. Neurological examination is also normal including reflexes, fundi, visual fields and motor power. Urine stick test is normal with no sugar.

Questions

- What possible differential diagnoses go through your mind?
- Should you refer him on to a specialist urologist?
- What advice can you give him?

ANSWER 47

Erectile dysfunction can be caused by cardiovascular problems (e.g. vascular disease in diabetes) reducing blood flow to the area, but the fact that this man can sustain an erection at other times, and the normal cardiovascular examination, make this unlikely. There is no evidence that he has low testosterone. Visual field defects are absent and there is no evidence of raised intracranial pressure or brain pathology. Smoking and alcohol consumption can affect sexual function. This is not obviously present but it will be worth asking more questions about potential illicit drug use or use of any other medications (neuroleptics and antihypertensives would be the usual culprits). Nervous system disorders that affect sexual function tend to be those affecting older people such as Parkinson's disease, cerebrovascular accident or multiple sclerosis, although trauma to the spine may also affect function. All of these are ruled out here by history and examination. Some local cancers or local disease (e.g. Peyronie disease) can be ruled out by normal appearance and the absence of pain or other symptoms. Aggressive cancer treatment or treatments for some systemic diseases can also affect erectile function.

There is no evidence of any physical illness. A referral to a urologist is likely to make him more anxious and is unnecessary at this point. The most likely diagnosis is that this man's problems are psychological. He is able to sustain a normal erection when he is not with his wife and he clearly has a high level of performance anxiety. This has been reinforced by experiences of premature ejaculation. Research shows that problems such as this can be greatly reduced by reduction in anxiety about performance.

In the first instance a lot of reassurance will help, as well as some literature to help him understand how the body works sexually and about different sexual needs within relationships. It will also help to explain the importance of the mind, expectations and circumstances in sexual relationships, and various self-help books may help him here. If these strategies do not work then he should return to you for other alternatives. It could be helpful to talk with him and his spouse together since it is difficult to fully understand the problems of one person in the relationship when sexuality is often expressed in a dynamic between two people. Discuss this option with him but respect his wishes. The attitudes and expectations of his wife may be relevant, and the solution may need to involve them both. It may be that a local couple's therapy or psychosexual clinic would help them. In this case, for example, it may be helpful to take the performance of sexuality out of the equation and ask them to explore each other's bodies through massage and caressing with an instruction not to have intercourse. It may be that mutual masturbation (if acceptable to them culturally) will allow him to see that he can maintain erection and reduce subsequent performance anxiety. Exploring sexuality together will also allow them as a couple to better understand each other's needs and preferences.

Many people's problems disappear with time and reassurance. A request to visit you again should the problem persist would allow you to review the situation and make a referral to a psychosexual clinic for support, if the problem does not resolve with reassurance and information.

Key Points

- Many people are anxious about sexual performance, especially in a new relationship.
- Simple advice and reassurance may be effective, with follow-up should the situation not improve with time.
- A psychosexual clinic can sometimes be helpful if problems persist.

CASE 48: I LOVE HIM BUT I DON'T WANT SEX

A 23-year-old woman presents with her new husband. He states that they had been dating for 2 years and his girlfriend had expressed a preference to wait to consummate their relationship until after marriage. They did this but since marriage she has clearly been reluctant for sex and is fearful of it. He explains that he is happy to be patient but has become increasingly concerned that she views any physical affection by him as pressure by him to engage in sexual activity. They have both felt that this issue is affecting other aspects of their relationship. The husband has had previous sexual relationships and denies any problems. The woman appears anxious about these discussions.

When you see the woman alone, she confesses that she has had two sexual relationships in the past. Both were 'horrible' experiences and in both relationships she did not feel her needs were met. She found the sex uncomfortable and on occasions painful. The second boyfriend had described her as 'frigid'. She was relieved when her current partner accepted that they would refrain from sex until after marriage. She has not discussed her previous experiences with her husband. She recalls feeling very uncomfortable with a friend of her father who had made suggestive remarks when she was about 18 and had just had her first sexual relationship. Her parents are very religious and she was brought up to believe that sex before marriage was not acceptable. They rarely talked about it, and always switched the television over if there were any sexual or intimate scenes of any kind.

The woman feels that sexual issues aside, the relationship with her husband is good. She finds her own responses to his displays of affection upsetting as she can understand why he finds it hurtful. She says that she would like to have a sex life, but she finds herself becoming very fearful and sometimes when her husband is being physically affectionate in bed, it makes her feel almost like 'she is being raped', even though he has never forced himself on her, and he always leaves her alone when she makes it clear she does not want sexual contact. She cannot explain this thought and wishes it was not there so that she could relax and enjoy their relationship. She wonders if having such a strong moral upbringing has made her regard sex as 'bad'. She works as a retail assistant and is happy in her job. There is no medical history of note. She drinks socially and does not smoke. She has not taken any illicit drugs.

Mental state examination

She presents as anxious but is open and communicative especially when seen alone. She describes herself as reasonably happy although is finding the current issue stressful. There is no deliberate self-harm ideation or any evidence of psychosis.

Physical examination

She tenses up when a vaginal examination is suggested but once reassured settles. There is nothing abnormal to find on examination.

Questions

- What are the types of sexual dysfunction that women may experience?
- What is the problem that this patient most likely has?
- What are the causes of sexual dysfunction in women?
- What are the appropriate treatment options?

ANSWER 48

In a relationship, discrepancies between the parties in sexual desire are common and usually worked through until an equilibrium is reached. It could be cyclical and related to periods, or related to changes in life events (e.g. having a baby), and these are usually dealt with supportively as part of the normal ebb and flow in the course of every relationship. Some couples present with greater problems than this.

Lack of arousal or desire may be temporary or ongoing. This may lead to difficulty becoming aroused or having an orgasm. In other cases, the woman feels sexual desire but cannot become aroused. Orgasm may not occur or may take a long time. In the latter case this usually simply requires the couple to understand this. This may be related to mood, atmosphere, timing, privacy or foreplay and all of these things can be adjusted if couples communicate with each other. If orgasm does not occur, many women get pleasure from love-making in other ways (caressing, intimacy, etc.). Some may get distressed and frustrated, especially if desire heightens without release. It can create a vicious cycle in which the woman loses interest in sex because the experience is not pleasurable.

Anorgasmia may be caused by the factors described above, hormonal problems, depression, bereavement or systemic illnesses, and these can all be addressed. Sometimes there can be no discernible cause.

Lack of desire or fear of sex can also be related to myriad different problems. There may be pain during intercourse (dyspareunia). This may be because of vaginal inflammation or dryness, vaginismus, endometriosis or pelvic inflammatory disease. A cause for this should be sought and treated. Side-effects from medication such as neuroleptics, chemotherapeutic agents and cardiovascular medication can affect arousal. Psychological morbidity can affect sexual functioning including depression, obsessive-compulsive disorder, anxiety and drug or alcohol abuse. Guilt, stress and resentment can all affect a woman's sexual function. Difficulties in an aspect of the relationship such as financial pressures, stresses of combining work and home life and childrearing issues may also be at play. Many people, either because of the way they were brought up or because of earlier bad experiences, do not view sex as a healthy part of a couple's relationship. Either partner may have unrealistic expectations about sex or make unreasonable requests. If the relationship is not good (e.g. if it involves fear or lack of mutual support) intimacy may be unwanted. Domestic violence would be an extreme example. History of abuse may lead to strong emotional negative responses to sexual intimacy or a lack of sufficient trust in her partner to relax and become aroused.

This woman should not be regarded as being ill, but may have a problem with fear of sexuality. It is important to make sure that the woman herself wants help and that she remains in control of her own body. If she does, this should be forthcoming without stigma.

Counselling is the first line of treatment. This will help the woman consider her previous experiences (both of sex and her upbringing) that are factors in the current presentation. The goal is to deal with attitudes that hinder her ability to view sex as enjoyable, establishing new attitudes that increase healthy sexual experiences. A sex therapist may take couples therapy one step further by focusing on the couple's physical relationship. After identifying the couple's attitudes about sex and the sexual problem, the sex therapist recommends specific exercises to re-focus the couple's attention and expectations. Group therapy or specialized support groups may allow a woman to discuss her problems with others who share them. Women often gain insight and practical solutions from these groups, as well as a greater confidence from knowing they are not alone.

Key Points

- Sexual problems of an acute or chronic nature are common.
- Physical causes need to be excluded.
- Sensitive and careful history taking is important.

CASE 49: HEROIN ADDICTION

History

A 19-year-old young man is brought to the general practitioner surgery by his sister with complaints of nausea, vomiting, body ache, fever, shivering and poor sleep over the past 2 days. He complains of having the 'flu' but his sister is worried that his symptoms may be related to drug use. He normally lives with his parents but is visiting her for the weekend. She says that he began smoking at the age of 14 and was using cannabis at age 16. He used to sniff glue at age 17 and was dabbling with opiates. Initially, he started smoking but then graduated to intravenous injections. He has been arrested twice for possession of Class A drugs and given cautions. His sister is extremely concerned about him. He denies using drugs in the presence of his sister. He says that he has experienced withdrawal having been without opiates for 48 hours when he could not find a dealer locally. Over the past few years the cost of his habit with heroin has increased from £20 a week to £300 per week. He admits that the drug clinic was not successful and that he now injects heroin twice a day. He enjoys the rush that he gets, but equally knows that he has needed to use more of the drug to achieve the same effect. He had enrolled in a youth training scheme but dropped out. He now has a rather fixed routine whereby he spends the day at home watching DVDs then going out later in the day with his friends for 'a fix'. He acknowledges that he ought to be 'getting out there' trying to get a job but said he did not have the confidence to do so as he had made several unsuccessful attempts at quitting. He does not abuse alcohol though he smokes 20 cigarettes a day. He gets unemployment benefits and says that he borrows money to fund his drug habit.

Mental state examination

He appears as a sullen, lanky young man, reluctant to talk. He speaks slowly but coherently, and there is no evidence of any psychotic symptoms. He appears tired and is yawning repeatedly. His mood appears anxious, and there is distinct psychomotor agitation. He has some insight into his substance misuse but presently begs to be prescribed some codeine or morphine for instant relief.

Physical examination

He has injection track marks in his cubital veins. His blood pressure is 148/98 mm Hg and pulse is 94 beats per minute, regular. His pupils appear dilated. He complains of muscle tenderness, but there is no significant finding on systemic examination.

Questions

- What is the differential diagnosis?
- What is the management plan?
- His sister is anxious to know what causes 'drug addiction' and wants to know what she can do to help. What will you tell her?

ANSWER 49

This young man meets the *International Classification of Diseases, Tenth Revision* (*ICD-10*) criteria for dependence syndrome (in this case opiates) based on the following criteria: (1) strong desire or compulsion to take the substance, (2) difficulty in controlling substance-use behavior, (3) physiological withdrawal on discontinuation of or reduction of substance intake, (4) evidence of tolerance (need for increasing doses of medication to achieve the initial effect of the drug), (5) progressive neglect of other interests and (6) persistence with substance use despite evidence of harmful consequences. Narrowing of the personal repertoire of pattern of substance misuse (e.g. always injecting with friends as opposed to at home) is also present.

Currently, however, he seems to be in opiate withdrawal.

! Symptoms and signs of opiate withdrawal

- Autonomic symptoms such as sweating, nausea, vomiting, diarrhoea, rhinorrhoea, lacrimation, shivering and piloerection ('cold turkey' refers to piloerection, or 'gooseflesh')
- Body aches or abdominal cramps
- Significant craving for opiates
- Central nervous system arousal such as sleeplessness, psychomotor agitation and tremors
- Repeated yawning

Heroin withdrawal typically peaks within 36–48 hours after discontinuation but symptoms persist for 7–14 days. Viral or bacterial gastroenteritis, acute pancreatitis, peptic ulcer or intestinal obstruction may mimic moderate to severe opioid withdrawal and need to be excluded as do psychiatric diagnoses such as mania, agitated depression and panic disorder. Co-morbid substance misuse is common, and withdrawal from benzodiazepines and alcohol (tremulousness, delirium and seizures) or intoxication with substances such as amphetamines (sympathetic overactivity) must also be considered.

Detailed history, mental state examination, physical examination for needle marks and appropriate investigations (urine toxicology screen, complete blood count and electrolyte levels) help clarify the diagnosis. He needs to be admitted to hospital to monitor his haemodynamic status, pupil size and bowel sounds. Opioid withdrawal is treated either by substitution with a long-acting opioid such as methadone or symptomatically with medications such as clonidine and benzodiazepines. He should be monitored closely for signs of continued illicit drug use. Psychological support and treatment of any co-morbid psychiatric illness ('dual diagnosis') are vital to improve long-term outcome.

His sister's concerns need to be addressed with an explanation of the biopsychosocial factors involved in aetiology. Opioid agonists act on μ-receptors rapidly producing physical dependence with strong reinforcement due to their euphoric effects. Gene polymorphisms have been implicated but environmental factors play a stronger role in causation. Social factors such as inner-city living, unemployment and poor parental functioning may play a role in initiation of drug use which is then maintained by reward conditioning. Psychological factors such as peer culture, education disenfranchisement and personality traits of curiosity and rebelliousness may also be related to initiation of drug use. Compassionate support without frustration even in the face of relapses, encouraging attendance at groups such as Narcotics Anonymous and support for family through self-help groups are likely to positively influence the outcome.

Key Points

- Sudden discontinuation of opioid intake in opiate-dependent individuals precipitates withdrawal, usually requiring inpatient assessment and treatment.
- Family support and psychological support are key to long-term cure.

CASE 50: EXHIBITIONISM

History

A 26-year-old carpet fitter presents to the emergency department having become embroiled in a fight. He says that a woman's boyfriend hit out at him for no reason. However, the paramedics report that the man had apparently 'flashed at the girlfriend and may have been masturbating'. Her boyfriend had sought to find out what was happening and a fight had started. The patient insists that he did not do anything inappropriate. When asked directly how he explains the other versions of events, he finally acknowledges that perhaps he had accidentally exposed his genitals. He then insists that this has never happened before, but when he is told that the police are waiting to interview him, he confesses he has been cautioned once before. He then states that he feels that he is not in control of himself and feels compelled to expose himself. He describes a tension that builds up inside him and a sense of relief when he has exposed. He admits that he has gradually exposed more on each occasion.

Mental state examination

His eye contact is furtive, but intermittently good. He is slightly agitated and appears anxious about the police wanting to interview him. His speech is normal. There are no signs of intoxication and his breath does not smell of alcohol. He is despondent in mood in the context of today's events, but there is no evidence to suggest depression. He can enjoy himself, holds down a job and has plans for his future. He does not have any hallucinations, thought disorder or delusions. He is orientated in time, place and person. There is no cognitive impairment.

A neurological examination is normal.

Questions

- What are the differential diagnoses?
- What is the most likely diagnosis?
- How would this be managed?

ANSWER 50

Several differential diagnoses should be considered. Organic conditions that may lead to disinhibition (such as drug and alcohol use, dementia or a space-occupying lesion) should be excluded. Organic causes are unlikely here given the history and normal neurological examination, although taking a fuller drug and alcohol history or obtaining a history about recent illness or behaviour from next of kin may be helpful. It is important to exclude exhibitionism as a presenting symptom in schizophrenia and affective disorder, especially mania where disinhibition is common. Some people with learning disabilities or Asperger syndrome may develop inappropriate sexually related behaviours. This may be through poor education or inappropriate channelling of sexual feelings and frustrations. A psychoeducational approach with support and reinforcement for healthy behaviours is often productive here. This man is not learning disabled (some clinicians and/or researchers use the term 'intellectual disability' in place of 'learning disability'), although some judicious questions to exclude autism spectrum disorder may be warranted. Exhibitionism can also occur without a mental illness and may or may not be related to antisocial personality disorder.

Exhibitionism is the exposure of one's genitals to a stranger, usually with no intention of further sexual activity with the other person. In some cases, the exhibitionist masturbates while exposing himself (or while fantasizing that he is exposing himself). Some exhibitionists are aware of a conscious desire to shock or upset their target, while others fantasize that the target will become sexually aroused by their display. Several theories have been proposed regarding the origins of exhibitionism but there is no established aetiology. Almost all reported cases involve males, but this may have much to do with gender and societal behaviours in that there is less censure when women expose themselves. Exposure for subcultural reasons (e.g. naturism) or for a bet (e.g. streaking) have different psychosocial meaning.

You need a thorough history (including sexual behaviours), mental state and neurological examination to rule out head trauma, seizures or other abnormalities of brain structure and function. Blood and urine tests for substance abuse and sexually transmitted diseases, including an HIV screen, should be considered.

Cognitive behaviour therapy is generally regarded as the most effective form of psychotherapy for exhibitionism. Group therapy when used needs to be done in an expert way to avoid reinforcing or perpetuating the thrill that the perpetrators may experience in discussion. Couples therapy or family therapy can be used if these relationships have been damaged, and if therapy is likely to be reparative. Social skills training and education will be helpful in learning disabilities and autism spectrum disorder. Medications such as selective serotonin reuptake inhibitors (SSRIs) can be tried if there is a strong obsessive-compulsive component. In some deviant sexual behaviours where there is a risk to others and psychosocial therapies have not worked, then assessment for hormonal interventions may be warranted. Consented surgery such as castration is usually reserved only for very serious and repeat sexual offenders.

The prognosis depends on several factors, including the age of onset, the reasons for the patient's referral to psychiatric care, degree of cooperation with the therapist and co-morbidity with other paraphilias (psychosexual disorders) or other mental disorders. People with exhibitionism have the highest recidivism rate of all the paraphilias. Recognition of paraphilias in adolescents and treatment for those at risk could lower the risk of recidivism.

Key Points

- Exhibitionism is one of a range of paraphilias.
- Treatment is difficult, and recidivism is high.

CASE 51: IRRITABLE, AGGRESSIVE AND ON A MISSION

History

A 22-year-old young man is admitted to a psychiatric inpatient unit under mental health legislation (e.g. Section 2 of the Mental Health Act in England). On admission, he is extremely agitated and hostile. He is very upset about having been admitted. He believes that he is of royal descent and is determined to punish those who are involved in 'imprisoning' him. It is reported by his family that he has no actual royal lineage, but that he sees himself as the person chosen to establish a new world government. He says he is on a mission. He has been angry and physically aggressive towards family members who contradict him. His grandmother banged the back of her head from when the man pushed her against a wall and has a bruised face. He refuses to allow a detailed mental status examination. He is pacing up and down the ward intimidating other patients. He is laughing out loud, talking to himself. He repeatedly makes threatening gestures at the ward staff.

He lives with his grandmother. He has no contact with his father. His mother died of a drug overdose when he was 6 years old. He uses cannabis regularly spending £20 a week but does not abuse alcohol or any other drugs. He smokes 40 cigarettes a day. There is no significant previous medical or psychiatric history. He has been behaving strangely, according to his grandmother, for the past 2 weeks. She has observed him spending a lot of money and talking openly about his sexual exploits to her. He has hardly slept over the past week. Two days ago, he threatened her and pushed her when she tried to urge him to see the doctor. Since then, she has been feeling increasingly frightened of him. He was prescribed the antipsychotic medication olanzapine 5 mg nocte (at night), which he has taken a few nights. However, this morning, he hit her. She reported the matter to the police, which ultimately led to his admission.

Mental state examination

He appears dishevelled bearing 3-day-old stubble. He is pacing imperiously up and down the ward corridor, singing out loud. He also laughs and talks to himself. Any attempts to interview him result in him swearing, and when he does agree to temporarily come into the interview room he very quickly walks out slamming the door as he goes. He gives little eye contact and appears preoccupied with his own thoughts. It is not possible to discuss his thoughts or experiences with him.

Physical examination

He refuses a physical examination.

Question

- How will you manage him?

ANSWER 51

This man is presenting with acute agitation, aggression and grandiose delusions. This may be an acute manic or psychotic episode, though an organic disorder or a drug-induced episode needs to be borne in mind. The immediate problem is containment of agitation and violence. National Institute for Health and Care Excellence (NICE) guidance advocates a three-step approach.

Risk assessment should be a continuous process to evaluate current risk and predict future risk. In this case, the risk for violence and aggression seems high as this man has several risk factors – a recent history of violence, current psychotic symptoms, continuing agitation, history of drug use, young age and male gender. He is irritable and has been threatening staff. Maintaining personal safety is a vital part of this risk assessment as is obtaining other information that informs this risk assessment. This may include general practitioner notes, corroborative history from his grandmother and medical and nursing records. Any advance directives by the patient must be taken into account.

Prevention of violence using *de-escalation* involves calming disruptive behaviour, giving clear choices and respecting dignity. Nursing observation levels should promote therapeutic engagement. Four levels are commonly used – general open, intermittent observation, within eyesight and within arm's length.

Interventions include physical intervention, seclusion and rapid tranquillization. Physical intervention – *control and restraint* – can compromise the patient's breathing and should be used sparingly only when necessary and by trained staff to safely immobilize an individual at immediate risk. *Seclusion*, the supervised confinement of a patient in a (usually locked) room, is to be used only as a last resort to ensure both the patient and staff are safe in severely disturbed behaviour. *Rapid tranquillization* is preferable to other physical interventions. Follow the local protocol. When agitation is *non-psychotic* or there is cardiovascular risk history, a short-acting benzodiazepine such as lorazepam is the first-choice medication. Commence with 2 mg orally, if required, repeated after at least 30 minutes. If oral medication is not accepted, intramuscular (IM) medication may be used beginning with a dose of 1 mg, repeated if required with 2 mg after at least 30 minutes. Maximum daily dose should not exceed 6 mg. Diazepam is long acting and has poor IM absorption and should therefore be avoided. The major tranquillizers olanzapine Velotab (5–10 mg maximum/24 hours) or haloperidol (5 mg oral, maximum 30 mg/d) may be added if there is no improvement with benzodiazepine alone. When *psychotic* agitation is present as in this case, a combination of lorazepam 1–2 mg oral with haloperidol 5–10 mg or with olanzapine 5–10 mg oral may be offered, repeated if required after at least 30 minutes. If offered as an IM dose, separate syringes must be used. IM lorazepam must not be given within 1 hour of IM olanzapine. Seek senior advice early, and all through this process monitor the patient's pulse, temperature, blood pressure and respiratory rate regularly (every 5–10 minutes until the patient is calm and ambulatory and hourly after that). Risk of cardiac arrest or respiratory depression is increased by physical agitation, by physical interventions and by drugs used in rapid tranquillization. Resuscitation expertise and equipment must be nearby.

Key Points

- Always use de-escalation as the preferred strategy to manage violence.
- Follow local rapid tranquillization protocol policy when using medication.

CASE 52: WHAT HAPPENS WHEN HE'S 18?

History

A young man a few months short of his 18th birthday is presented to his general practitioner (GP) in a state of agitation. Although his parents are worried about him, he does not really think there is a problem. He is hearing voices that are auditory hallucinations and these cause him some anxiety. The voices sometimes give a running commentary of what is happening. He denies any substance misuse. He attended Child and Adolescent Mental Health Services (CAMHS) about 12 months ago when he had lost interest in his previous activities and had become increasingly withdrawn although no low mood was reported. He was lost to follow-up when his family sent him to live with some relatives in the hope that a new environment might improve the situation. He has recently returned home but the situation is worsening rather than improving.

Questions

- What is the possible diagnosis?
- What are the challenges this young man's age presents?

ANSWER 52

The differential diagnoses in this case are schizophrenia, substance-induced psychosis and depression with psychosis. Schizophrenia is the most likely diagnosis. It is highly likely that he was in the prodromal phase of the illness when he first presented.

The risk is that this young man may fall between two services. Transition is a time of change from one place/service to another. Most CAMHS provide care to young people up to their 18th birthday. He is soon going to be too old for CAMHS, and his care will need to be transferred to adult mental health services (AMHS). The risk is exacerbated by the fact that he does not have much insight and so engagement with one (let alone two) services may be difficult for him.

Examples of mental health problems and how transition unfolds include

- Transition to AMHS and remaining with those services because of enduring mental illness such as schizophrenia
- Transition to AMHS and subsequently dropping out of services (some eating disorders may fall into this category)
- Referral to AMHS but not accepted for a service. (For many cases of autism spectrum disorder and attention deficit hyperactivity disorder (ADHD) there are no adult services available. Increasingly more adult services for adult ADHD are being commissioned, but these may still not be present in many places.)
- Not needing to move to adult services if CAMHS could work with them for longer. (Some disorders such as an episode of depression may be treated for a while after the 18th birthday to offer continuity of care.)
- Not needing to move to adult services as the problems are resolved before the need for transfer of care. (For example episodes of depression, obsessive-compulsive disorder and anxiety may fall in this group although many of these may recur in adulthood.)

For those young people who do continue to have severe mental health problems that require a transition to AMHS, this transition from one service to another should be a smooth process that offers uninterrupted continuity of care.

There can be differences between CAMHS and AMHS in relation to thresholds regarding acceptance criteria, professional differences and service structures/configurations which affect the transition process. CAMHS and AMHS services often take differing approaches in the ways in which they work.

To improve transitions there should be

- Joint policies between services
- Local commissioning arrangements that avoid service gaps
- National and local policy documents describing models of care (e.g. preventative strategies, agreed guidelines for treatment, etc.)
- Local transition agreements that are described in service specifications (e.g. joint appointments 1 year before service move)

Key Points

- Special care needs to be taken at transitions to ensure vulnerable patients are not lost to follow-up.
- There is a need for CAMHS and AMHS to place the young person at the centre of care.
- Given that CAMHS and AMHS may work in different ways, there is a need to ensure that the concerns of the parents are heard and appropriate support provided for them, too.

CASE 53: THOUGHTS OF KILLING HER BABY

History

A 28-year-old mother of a 2-month-old baby boy attends the general practitioner (GP) surgery having been referred by her health visitor as she had become concerned about the safety of the baby following a routine postnatal check-up. The mother says that she is finding it difficult to cope with the baby and sometimes has had thoughts that it would have been better if the baby was dead. She has feelings of guilt about having such thoughts and believes that she is not a good mother. The baby was born at full term via a normal vaginal delivery. The labour lasted 18 hours and there were no other complications. She reported feeling low and tearful during the first week post-partum but said that her mood improved within a few days. However, over the past 6 weeks, she describes feeling low and tired all the time. She complains of low energy levels, poor concentration and does not enjoy looking after her son as much as she did in the past. She feels overwhelmed with the responsibility of looking after the baby and has lost her self-confidence. Her sleep is poor.

She works as a nurse in a local hospital and went off work at 32 weeks of pregnancy. She was treated for a depressive episode by her GP 4 years ago. She had been prescribed fluoxetine 20 mg once a day. She took the medication for a year and then stopped the medication as she felt better. There is no other psychiatric or medical history. Her parents are retired and live in a different city. Her mother suffers from recurrent depressive disorder and has been treated with electroconvulsive therapy (ECT) in the past.

This is her first child and it was a planned pregnancy. She lives with her husband who is an engineer. She describes herself as a perfectionist who likes doing things in a particular way. She is a non-smoker and a social drinker.

Mental state examination

This woman is seen by her GP at home. She is dressed in her night clothes, has greasy hair and has not taken a shower. She is holding the baby appropriately but does not smile or make eye contact with the baby. During the interview she bottle feeds the baby. She has discontinued breastfeeding due to mastitis. She feels that she has let her baby down by not being able to breastfeed. She speaks in a monotonous voice and becomes tearful when asked how she is coping. She has feelings of guilt about not being a good mother. She says that she has had thoughts that it would be better if the baby was dead. On one occasion an image of her putting a pillow over the baby's face flashed through her mind, although she says she would never do this. She finds these thoughts distressing. She has thoughts of wanting to be dead but does not have any definite suicidal plans. Cognitive examination did not reveal any impairment.

Questions

- What is the differential diagnosis?
- How would you manage this patient?

ANSWER 53

This woman is suffering from postnatal depression, which is defined as depression occurring after childbirth. It is seen most often within 4 weeks of childbirth but can occur up to 6 months post-partum. The symptoms of postnatal depression are similar to those seen in a depressive disorder. She has all the core symptoms of depression including low mood, low energy levels and anhedonia. These symptoms have been present for more than 2 weeks. She also has additional symptoms of depression such as feelings of guilt, loss of confidence, poor sleep and suicidal thoughts. She has had an episode of depression in the past and therefore fulfils the criteria for a recurrent depressive disorder, with the current episode being moderate to severe. The prevalence rate of postnatal depression is between 8% and 20%. Many such women have had depression in the past. It is important to screen for depression in pregnancy and health visitors can use the Edinburgh Postnatal Depression Scale (EPDS) as a part of antenatal check-up.

! Differential diagnosis

- *Post-partum blues* is seen in up to 75% of women and is characterized by a mild self-limiting episode of mood disturbance lasting a few days. It usually begins 3–10 days post-partum (peak onset days 5–7) and resolves spontaneously.
- *Post-partum psychosis* is seen in 1% of women and is characterized by rapid onset of labile mood, thought disorder, confusion and disorientation. Previous history and family history of mental illness, particularly of bipolar disorder, are significant risk factors. This is a severe disorder and often requires inpatient treatment. Delirium (e.g. infective) needs to be excluded with this presentation.

Management

This woman needs to be referred to a specialist Mother and Baby (Perinatal Psychiatric) team for urgent assessment of the risk of harm to the baby and risk of self-harm, which dictates the course of further management. One option, depending on risk and choice, is admission to the Mother and Baby Unit for further assessment and management. There are several benefits of admitting mother and baby together. It lets the mother continue to breastfeed, allows for healthy development of attachment and maintains the confidence of the mother in her parenting ability. Parenting assessment allows early detection of problems with attachment and institution of remedial measures. Treatment for the depression includes cognitive behaviour therapy (CBT) and/or pharmacotherapy. Lofepramine, fluoxetine and sertraline, although expressed in breast milk, are considered relatively safe, unlike medications such as lithium and sodium valproate which should not be used in breastfeeding mothers. If the parenting assessment raises concerns about the safety of the child (risk of harm or neglect), then a referral to the child safeguarding team should be made. Occasionally involuntary detention under the local Mental Health Act may be warranted especially if there is high risk and little insight from the mother.

Key Points

- Childbirth is a vulnerable period for women with risk of post-partum blues, post-partum depression and post-partum psychosis.
- Be aware of medications expressed in breast milk.
- Risk to the baby should dictate early involvement of specialist Mother and Baby Unit and child protection teams.
- Health visitors and GPs need to have a high index of suspicion.

CASE 54: MY WIFE IS HAVING AN AFFAIR

History

A 45-year-old publican presents to his general practitioner (GP) complaining of being unable to cope with his wife's behaviour. He goes on to tell the GP that his wife of over 20 years has recently begun to have numerous affairs with customers at the pub they run. He can tell whom his wife has had an affair with because of the 'way she looks at them'. He has confronted her about this on several occasions but she denies his accusations. As a result of his suspicions, he keeps a log of the mileage of her car to check where she has been. His wife has become very upset by the change in his behaviour and has moved into the spare bedroom. He has taken this as further confirmation that she is having an affair.

He first became concerned about his wife's behaviour a month ago. Since that time his mood has been low and he has become increasing preoccupied by thoughts of her infidelity. His sleep, appetite and concentration are poor. He has begun to have financial problems as he is finding it hard to run the public house due to the stress he is under.

He has previously suffered from moderate depressive episodes and stopped his anti-depressant medication over a year ago. There is no other past medical or psychiatric history of note. He describes himself as a 'social drinker' due to his job. On direct questioning he admits to a gradual increase in his alcohol intake over the last couple of years. He is now drinking every day and typically consumes in excess of 60 units per week. There is no history of illicit substance abuse.

Mental state examination

He has good eye contact and is perspiring. He presents as an overweight middle-aged man who is slightly unkempt and smells of alcohol. He is initially reluctant to talk about his difficulties, repeatedly saying that his wife would not be having affairs if he was 'a real man'. He reports that his mood is 'terrible' and objectively he appears low. His thought content is mainly concerned with the belief that his wife is being unfaithful. He is unwilling to even accept the possibility that he may be mistaken, yet has no concrete evidence upon which he has reached this conclusion. There is no abnormality of perception and his cognition is grossly intact. He does not think he is mentally unwell but is willing to accept help to deal with the stress he is under.

Physical examination

The only abnormality upon physical examination is palmar erythema and mild hepatomegaly.

Questions

- What term is used to describe this presentation?
- What is the differential diagnosis for this presentation?
- Who may be at risk from this patient?

ANSWER 54

This patient falsely believes that his wife is being unfaithful. He has reached this conclusion in the absence of any appropriate evidence and despite evidence to the contrary. He holds this belief with absolute conviction, and he is becoming increasingly preoccupied by this belief. This presentation is often referred to as pathological jealousy (also known as morbid jealousy or Othello syndrome). Pathological jealousy is a descriptive term rather than a diagnosis and its differential diagnosis is shown in the following box.

Differential diagnosis of pathological jealousy

- Depressive episode with psychotic symptoms: evidence of sustained low mood with decreased sleep, appetite and concentration. Psychotic symptoms are in keeping with low mood (i.e. mood congruent).
- Delusional disorder: presence of delusional beliefs with an absence of other symptoms such as hallucinations.
- Schizophrenia: presence of delusions and hallucinations with an absence of prominent mood symptoms.
- Schizoaffective disorder: mood and psychotic symptoms are equally prominent but psychotic symptoms may not be in keeping with the expressed mood (i.e. mood incongruent).
- Organic psychosis: may be due to alcohol/illicit substance abuse or underlying physical disorder such as brain tumour or temporal lobe epilepsy (TLE).
- Paranoid personality disorder: lifelong pattern of suspicion of the motives of others with a tendency to misperceive neutral events as hostile and threatening.
- Asperger syndrome with misinterpretation of the motives of others.

Those with pathological jealousy are distressed by their false belief in their partner's infidelity and show unreasonable behaviour (such as checking for proof that their partner is being unfaithful and frequent accusations). This can escalate to become increasingly extreme. This combination of strong emotions and acting upon delusional beliefs is particularly dangerous. The patient's partner may be at increased risk, and the risk of homicide in such situations can be high. A referral to adult safeguarding or the police may be necessary. Other people could also be at risk from the patient if he believes that they are involved in his partner's infidelity. Breaching the patient's confidentiality in the interest of public safety may be justified. Finally, the patient himself is at increased risk of suicide due to the high level of distress and conviction that his partner is being unfaithful. These risks will be further increased in the presence of alcohol/illicit substance abuse.

Key Points

- Pathological jealousy is a descriptive term, not a diagnosis, and a careful assessment should be made to obtain an underlying diagnosis.
- Those presenting with these symptoms may pose a risk to themselves, their partners and others. Co-morbid substance misuse is often present and further increases the risk of harm to others and self.
- A detailed risk assessment must be conducted in all cases of pathological jealousy.

CASE 55: A MAN IN POLICE CUSTODY

History

A 20-year-old roofer is brought to the emergency department by the police. He is under arrest after having been charged with assaulting his girlfriend. They had both been drinking and then had an argument during which he punched her several times. During the ensuing struggle he fell and struck his head on the kerb. Following this he was unresponsive for a few seconds. When the police arrived he was alert and denied any physical problems. While in the police van, on the way to the police station, he vomited and appeared to become unresponsive for approximately 30 seconds.

In the custody cell, he is loudly shouting and swearing at the accompanying police officers. On attempting to get a history, he becomes more agitated, repeatedly shouting, 'I know what you're here for. They want you to give me a lethal injection'.

He is normally fit and well and has no previous history of psychiatric disorder or substance abuse. The accompanying police officers say that he has not been previously known to the police.

Mental state examination

He presents as a slim, reasonably kempt young man who smells of alcohol. He is agitated and restless, and eye contact is variable. He is difficult to engage and answers most questions by being verbally abusive. After some persuasion, he eventually acknowledges that he is being offered help and he agrees to cooperate with the assessment. His speech is loud, rapid and slurred. He says that he is worried that the police might want to kill him and that he can see bats flying around the department. Upon cognitive testing he is able to correctly tell his name and date of birth but is not able to correctly state the current day, month or year. His short-term memory also appears to be impaired.

Physical examination

Cardiovascular, respiratory and abdominal examinations are normal. Upon neurological examination he has an up-going left plantar response but no other abnormality.

Questions

- What investigations would you want to carry out in this patient?
- The police and nurses tell you that he is 'just drunk' and request your advice about returning him to police custody as soon as you have finished your physical examination. What would be your response?

ANSWER 55

Although he appears intoxicated with alcohol and agitated following the argument with his girlfriend, there are several indicators of a possible organic cause for his current presentation (such as subdural haematoma). He has a history of having sustained a recent head injury that caused him to lose consciousness and since then he has vomited and had a further brief period of possible loss of consciousness. There is also a non-specific abnormality on neurological examination. His speech is slurred and he is agitated (although this could also be due to alcohol intoxication). In addition to this, he has psychotic symptoms (believing that the police want to kill him and seeing bats) and cognitive impairment (disorientated to time and impaired short-term memory) which are probably of acute onset. While visual hallucinations can occur in functional mental illnesses (such as schizophrenia) they are relatively rare and often indicate the presence of an underlying organic disorder. Given all these factors it is important to rule out any possible organic causes of this man's presentation by physical examination and appropriate use of investigations.

Investigations

- Obtain further collateral history: previous medical records (including psychiatric and general practitioner notes if available) and further information from the police and the patient's girlfriend/family.
- Urine illicit drug screen to exclude intoxication with drugs such as amphetamine or cannabis.
- Blood tests including full blood count (FBC), urea and electrolytes (U+Es), calcium, liver function tests (LFTs), thyroid function tests (TFTs) and C-reactive protein (CRP). The results of these tests will help to exclude infection or metabolic derangement.
- Computerized tomography (CT) brain scan to exclude cerebrovascular event (i.e. haemorrhage or infarction) or space-occupying lesion (i.e. tumour, subdural haematoma or abscess).

Given the high index of suspicion of an organic basis for this man's presentation, it is imperative that he does not leave the emergency department until this has either been excluded or he has received appropriate treatment. Your response to these requests should be to politely but firmly point out that there are some parts of this man's presentation that do not fit with a simple diagnosis of 'acute alcohol intoxication'. You should state that it is important he receives appropriate clinical care, based on the results of these investigations, to exclude other organic causes. If an organic cause is excluded and he is thought to be mentally ill, then he may be offered admission to an inpatient psychiatric unit. It will be important to assess whether he has the capacity to consent to admission, failing which, an involuntary admission may be required using the appropriate local capacity or mental health legislation (Mental Capacity Act and Mental Health Act, respectively, in England).

Key Points

- The acute onset of cognitive problems or psychotic symptoms (especially visual hallucinations) may indicate an acute organic condition.
- Always have a high index of suspicion for organic causes of 'psychiatric' presentations and employ appropriate physical examination and investigations to rule them out.
- Alcohol intoxication may mask the presence of underlying physical conditions.

CASE 56: STALKING

History

A 20-year-old mathematics student is referred by the university counselling service. He is currently suspended from his studies due to alleged harassment of a female student. He has been repeatedly sending this student text messages (over 20 per day for the last 6 months) and spends much of his day loitering around the halls of residence where she lives. He has told his family that he and the female student are engaged and that when they met, it was 'love at first sight'. The female student denies this, saying that she has never had a relationship with him, has no wish to do so and finds his behaviour towards her extremely upsetting. She has informed him on numerous occasions that she does not wish to have any contact with him. At the request of his tutor he was seen by the university counselling service. During the initial assessment he told the counsellor that he and the female student were in love and that he felt angry that she could not admit this and had reported him to the university. Since she did this his behaviour towards her has become more intense and he has had thoughts of killing her, saying that this would be the only way to maintain their 'pure love' without the interference of others.

He has always been a somewhat shy and introverted person and he has never previously had an intimate relationship. He has no personal or family history of psychiatric disorder. He is socially isolated and has few friends, preferring to spend his free time playing computer games. In the last 2 months he has been cautioned by the police regarding his behaviour towards the female student but has no previous convictions.

Mental state examination

He avoids eye contact and is difficult to engage. He speaks in a monotonous voice and becomes much more animated when discussing his love for the female student and his hobby of playing computer games. His mood appears normal and there have not been any recent changes in his sleep pattern or appetite. Throughout the interview he professes his love for the female student and says that this is mutual but that she cannot show others how she feels because they would be jealous of their 'special relationship'. He confirms that he has had intermittent thoughts of killing the female student as a way of maintaining their 'pure love'. There is no abnormality of perception and his cognition is normal.

Questions

- What psychiatric disorders may be associated with this presentation?
- How would you manage the risk he may pose to the female student?

ANSWER 56

This stalking behaviour may be due to erotomania (also known as de Clerambault syndrome) in which a person falsely believes, with delusional intensity, that another person is in love with him or her. Erotomania is a descriptive term rather than a diagnosis and some of its potential causes are as follows:

- Delusional disorder involves the presence of delusions with an absence of other psychopathology (i.e. no evidence of hallucinations or abnormality of mood).
- Schizophrenia will have evidence of hallucinations, thought disorder and delusions.
- Schizoaffective disorder has an equal presentation of schizophrenic and mood symptomatology.
- Hypomania includes evidence of disinhibited behaviour and grandiose beliefs.
- Organic disorders will show evidence of substance abuse or physical illness on physical examination.
- Schizoid personality disorder shows a long-standing pattern of avoidance of social situations, emotional coldness and social awkwardness.
- Schizotypal personality disorder has a long-standing pattern of odd behaviour and ideas with magical thinking and quasi-psychotic experiences.
- Autism spectrum disorder since early childhood evidence of impairment in social relationships and communication; often accompanied by a narrow, restricted range of interests and repetitive behaviour. Mind blindness means that they have difficulties understanding the emotions of others and frequently misinterpret their intentions and feelings.

The main management of erotomania is treatment of the underlying disorder. However, in cases such as these an assessment should be made of the risk that the patient may pose to others. The object of the patient's affection may be at particular risk and strong feelings of love may suddenly turn to feelings of frustration, grievance and hate if the patient feels his or her advances have been unfairly rejected. Other people may be at risk if the patient feels that they are somehow responsible for the failure of the 'relationship'.

In order to effectively manage this risk it may sometimes be necessary to involve other services/agencies such as the police, probation service and social services. Given that the patient may pose a particular risk to an identifiable individual, the issue of warning the person that he or she is potentially at risk should also be considered. Doing this may be a justifiable (and necessary) breach of medical confidentiality. This should only be done following discussion with a senior colleague and careful evaluation of the risks and benefits of disclosure and non-disclosure of this information.

Key Points

- Stalking behaviour may be a symptom of mental illness.
- The management of such individuals may be complex and require the involvement of several different agencies (e.g. psychiatric services, police, probation services and social services).
- Where there is evidence that a named individual may be at risk from the patient, consideration should be given to breaking confidentiality and informing this person.

CASE 57: AN ANGRY MAN

History

A 27-year-old unemployed man has been referred by his general practitioner (GP) for help with managing his anger. He has recently moved to the area and no previous medical or psychiatric notes are available. He tells you that he 'lives on his wits' but has just been released from prison 3 weeks ago.

As a child he had behavioural problems and was expelled from several different schools. He saw a child psychologist between the ages of 11 and 14 years. After leaving school at 15, with no qualifications, he has held a number of short-term unskilled jobs. He is always able to get jobs but has trouble keeping them because his short temper leads him to fall out with his colleagues. He says that he has a similar problem with relationships and admits that he has previously been violent towards his partners. He has had extensive contact with the criminal justice system and has spent much of the last 10 years in prison for offences including burglary, grievous bodily harm, driving while disqualified, benefit fraud and drugs offences. When discussing his previous offending he says that he was justified in doing this because he needed the money and that the people he assaulted deserved it and that he wishes he had caused them more injuries. He has a number of debts upon which he has defaulted payment. He tells you that his criminal behaviour is a failure of 'the system' and that he has been 'forced' into this lifestyle due to the failure of others to provide him with sufficient support.

He denies any other previous psychiatric history but as the interview progresses he asks if you can prescribe him benzodiazepines as he has been previously told by a 'top psychiatrist' that these are the only treatment that will help him. He has received treatment for a number of injuries received in 'fights' but denies any other past medical history. He is currently living in a bail hostel where he is under the supervision of the probation service. He has an extensive history of substance abuse that includes alcohol, cannabis, heroin and amphetamine, but says that he has managed to remain abstinent from these since being released from prison.

Mental state examination

He initially presents as appropriate and cooperative. His mood is euthymic and there is no evidence of delusions or hallucinations. He becomes defensive when asked about his previous contact with psychiatric services saying that it is 'none of your business'. When you decline to prescribe benzodiazepines he becomes angry and storms out of the room.

Questions

- Is there any evidence that this man is suffering from a personality disorder?
- If so what personality disorder is most likely?
- What features of this personality disorder does he display?

ANSWER 57

The evidence for this man having a personality disorder is that he displays evidence of behaviours, cognitions and emotions that cause problems for him and others around him. These difficulties are evident in a number of different situations and appear to have persisted throughout his life and began in childhood. It is most likely that he is suffering from dissocial personality disorder. This is an *International Classification of Diseases, Tenth Revision* (*ICD-10*) term; in the *Diagnostic and Statistical Manual of Mental Disorders, Fifth Edition* (*DSM-5*) a similar personality disorder is called *antisocial personality disorder* (APD). The features of this personality disorder are shown in the following box.

Features of dissocial (antisocial) personality disorder

- Evidence of Conduct Disorder before the age of 15 (required for *DSM-5* diagnosis of Antisocial Personality Disorder but not for *ICD-10* Dissocial Personality Disorder)
- Callous unconcern for the feelings of others
- Gross and persistent irresponsibility and disregard for social rules, norms and obligations
- Inability to form enduring relationships although has no difficulty in establishing them
- Low tolerance to frustration and easily becomes angry or aggressive
- Incapacity to experience guilt or profit from experience
- Marked proneness to blame others for his or her difficulties

Most people with this disorder do not seek psychiatric treatment. Patients with dissocial personality disorder are often challenging to manage and can evoke strong negative feelings in others. Recognizing these feelings (counter-transference) is important and helps in establishing and maintaining a therapeutic relationship. As would be expected from the clinical features, they are at increased risk of engaging in criminality and violence. They are also at increased risk of death from suicide, accidents and violence.

A diagnosis of dissocial personality disorder does not absolve an individual of responsibility for any criminal acts that he or she commits. The criminal justice system (police, prisons, courts and probation service) frequently manage such individuals (although they may not necessarily be labelled as having this disorder). It is important to maintain clear boundaries and rules when treating these patients. Any associated criminal offending is often best managed by the criminal justice system rather than mental health services.

Key Points

- In order to make a diagnosis of personality disorder it is important to take a detailed history of the patient's difficulties throughout their lifetime and in different situations.
- Patients with dissocial personality disorder can arouse negative counter-transference. Recognizing this helps therapeutic engagement.
- The diagnosis of dissocial personality disorder does not absolve the patient of responsibility for any criminal acts he or she commits and the patient may be more appropriately managed by the criminal justice system.

CASE 58: THE TREATMENT ISN'T WORKING

History

A 38-year-old receptionist is referred by her general practitioner (GP) to the psychiatric outpatient clinic as she has failed to respond to two different antidepressants. She was well until 2 years ago when she started feeling very tired and found it difficult to concentrate at work. Over the next 6 months, she developed back pain and joint pains. Detailed investigations did not reveal any abnormality. She went on to develop anhedonia, restlessness, poor sleep and excessive appetite leading to a weight gain of 6 kg over 6 months. She was getting increasingly irritable at work and so was prescribed the serotonin reuptake inhibitor citalopram 20 mg daily by her GP. She took the tablets consistently but with no benefit. The dose was increased gradually up to 50 mg a day without any improvement. After nearly 4 months of treatment she had continued low mood, low energy and anhedonia. Citalopram was discontinued and replaced with the tetracyclic antidepressant mirtazapine. There was an initial marginal improvement in her tiredness and sleep, but this was transient. The dose of mirtazapine was increased up to 45 mg per day without any benefit.

She continues to attend work but feels tired and fed up all the time. She denies any ideas of self-harm, but acknowledges that most mornings she has thoughts that she would be better off dead. She had her appendix removed 5 years ago but has no other significant medical history. There is no previous psychiatric history of note. She lives with her boyfriend and their two cats in their own home. She reports reduced interest in sex, but apart from that has a happy relationship with her boyfriend. Her father left her mother when she was 3 years old. She has had no contact with her father since then. Her mother suffers from multiple sclerosis, but there is no other family history. She has one elder sister who is well. Pre-morbidly, she says that she was a happy-go-lucky person with no care in the world.

Mental state examination

Her eye contact is steady but she appears downcast and lethargic. Her speech is slow and soft though she gets somewhat agitated when talking about her father. Her mood is low and her affect reflects this. She describes ideas of hopelessness, helplessness and worthlessness. She does not have any ideas of self-harm. There is no evidence of any psychotic symptoms.

Questions

- What is the diagnosis?
- How would you manage this patient?

ANSWER 58

This woman is presenting with a 2-year history of low mood, reduced energy, anhedonia, reduced sleep and libido, weight gain and ideas of hopelessness, helplessness and worthlessness. If organic causes of depression are excluded she thus meets the criteria for a depressive episode. She has been treated with two different antidepressants (from different groups), using appropriate doses for an appropriate duration, but has not shown an adequate response. This suggests a treatment-resistant depressive episode. The definition of treatment-resistant depression (TRD) is somewhat arbitrary, but National Institute for Health and Care Excellence (NICE) guidance defines it as failure to return to a baseline mood state despite an adequate trial with at least two antidepressant medications. So defined, 20%–30% of patients with major depression are treatment resistant. The causes of treatment resistance may include

- Incorrect diagnosis: bipolar mood disorder, personality disorder, schizoaffective disorder, depression secondary to a medical disorder, adjustment disorder, persistent stress/trauma, or dual diagnosis with drug or alcohol misuse
- Inadequate treatment: inadequate dose or duration of treatment, poor compliance or incorrect choice of antidepressant therapy (e.g. not using electroconvulsive therapy [ECT] in catatonic depression)

! Antidepressant groups

- Selective serotonin reuptake inhibitors (SSRIs) (e.g. fluoxetine)
- Serotonin–noradrenaline reuptake inhibitors (SNRIs) (e.g. venlafaxine)
- Tricyclics (e.g. amitriptyline)
- Tertracyclics (e.g. mirtazapine)
- Monamine oxidase inhibitors (e.g. phenelzine)

This woman needs referral to specialist mental health services for management of her TRD. The suggested step-wise protocol for managing TRD is as follows:

- Review diagnosis and alter treatment as appropriate.
- Review possibility of lifestyle changes.
- Optimize antidepressant dose (monotherapy with SSRI, venlafaxine, tricyclic antidepressant [TCA] or mirtazapine).
- Ensure adequate duration of treatment.
- Optimize psychotherapy and social interventions where necessary. This may include considering alteration in individual therapy modality (e.g. cognitive behaviour therapy, interpersonal therapy, etc.), group or family therapy.
- Switch to another antidepressant class (monotherapy with SSRI, venlafaxine, TCA or mirtazapine).
- Switch to TCA, venlafaxine or monoamine oxidase inhibitor (MAOI).
- Consider augmentation with lithium.
- Consider use of antidepressant combinations that are least prone to toxicity and interactions (mianserin or mirtazapine with SSRI; TCA + SSRI; venlafaxine + SSRI, etc.). Monitor for the potentially fatal serotonin syndrome characterized by the triad of autonomic hyperactivity, neuromuscular dysfunction (tremors, myoclonic jerks) and mental confusion or delirium.
- Consider use of ECT.

In this case, venlafaxine or a TCA may be the next management step.

Key Points

- In cases of TRD, review diagnosis, dose, duration of treatment and co-morbidity (with alcohol, drugs or other psychiatric or medical disorder).
- Identify TRD early and refer to the specialist mental health service for management as per protocol above.

CASE 59: THE DRUGS AREN'T HELPING

History

A 26-year-old man is referred to the crisis intervention home treatment team by his community psychiatric nurse. He is interviewed at home in the presence of his wife and 3-year-old child. He has turned the house upside down as he is convinced that there is a microphone taping his family conversations. He has been hugging his child, crying inconsolably. He can hear some 'young lads down the road' talking about killing him and his family. He feels that TV programmes are discussing him and his family. He has taped newspapers on the windows and has set up trip wires at the front and back doors. He has not slept for 3 days and has been talking to himself. He was diagnosed with schizophrenia at the age of 20 and was under the care of the Early Intervention Team for 3 years. He was treated with risperidone and seemed to have responded well. However, he stopped taking his medication and had a relapse 2 years ago. He was assigned a community psychiatric nurse as his care coordinator. Risperidone was re-commenced but he continued to remain paranoid and suspicious. There was concern about the possibility of him missing medication, and he was switched to risperidone long-acting depot. This was continued for over 12 months but without a significant response. Risperidone was replaced with olanzapine but this also did not produce a significant response and was associated with weight gain of 3 stones. Olanzapine was discontinued 3 months ago and he was prescribed aripiprazole. His wife insists that he has been compliant, but over the last 6 weeks his mental state has deteriorated.

Mental state examination

He appears very frightened and agitated. His eyes are darting and he is cowering on the sofa clutching his daughter, who is calm but looks frightened. He seems to be responding to unseen stimuli and occasionally mutters to himself. He says that voices describe what he is doing in a commentary. His mood is labile and he breaks down repeatedly. His speech is coherent and relevant. There is no formal thought disorder but he has delusions of persecution and reference. He does acknowledge that he has mental illness, but feels frustrated that his suspicions are not being taken seriously.

Questions

- What is the diagnosis?
- What is the next step in pharmacological management?

ANSWER 59

This man is currently experiencing delusions of persecution and reference and auditory hallucinations. His symptoms have been present for nearly 2 years with significant worsening in the past 6 weeks. These symptoms have failed to respond to adequate doses of more than two different antipsychotics, thus meeting the criteria for treatment-resistant schizophrenia (TRS). About 10%–30% of patients do not respond to antipsychotics and a further 30% have only a partial response. However, before TRS is diagnosed: (1) review the diagnosis. Consider co-morbid disorders such as depression which may mimic treatment-resistant negative symptoms and medical disorders such as endocrine or neurological disorders. (2) Check whether there is co-morbid substance misuse that may contribute to treatment resistance. (3) Assess the dose, duration and compliance of drug treatment. Ensure that at least two antipsychotics (at least one of which is an atypical) have been used at appropriate doses for at least 6 weeks. (4) Consider whether psychosocial interventions appropriate to the stage of illness are in place.

Clozapine has been consistently shown to be effective in TRS, improving symptoms and quality of life, and is the only medication licensed for the treatment of TRS and to be recommended by National Institute for Health and Care Excellence (NICE) guidelines for this purpose. Despite its association with some serious side effects (see following), when prescribed with close monitoring (as occurs in the United Kingdom) it can be a safe and effective treatment.

- Neutropenia or potentially fatal agranulocytosis has been reported, so leucocytes and complete blood counts need to be monitored weekly for 18 weeks and then every 2 weeks up to a year, after which, if the blood counts are stable, they can be done 4-weekly. Clozapine must be discontinued immediately if leucocyte count is $<3000/mm^3$ or neutrophil count is $<1500/mm^3$. An urgent referral to a haematologist is needed. Clozapine should never be re-prescribed in such cases. Concomitant use of drugs that increase the risk of agranulocytosis such as carbamazepine and azapropazone should be avoided.
- Cardiomyopathy and fatal myocarditis (most commonly in the first 2 months) have been reported. Detailed history, physical examination and electrocardiogram (ECG) should be accompanied by close monitoring for persistent tachycardia in the first 2 months.
- Postural hypotension can lead to collapse and therefore clozapine should only be initiated in closely supervised settings such as an inpatient unit, day hospital or under the care of the home treatment team.
- Clozapine can reduce the seizure threshold, so drugs lowering the seizure threshold should be avoided. The risk of hypotension and seizures means that if the clozapine is missed for >48 hours due to non-concordance or vomiting, the dose must be re-titrated gradually commencing at 12.5 mg to 25 mg/d.
- Other side effects include sedation (slow dose titration), hypersalivation (treated with hyoscine), constipation (advocate fibre diet), weight gain and diabetes (monitor blood glucose, triglyceride levels, weight, body mass index and ECG prior to commencement and during treatment) and elevated liver enzymes (monitor liver function tests).

Plasma clozapine level is not monitored routinely but is useful in optimizing treatment and monitoring compliance. If TRS does not respond to clozapine, augmentation with another antipsychotic is recommended. All this must occur alongside psychosocial treatments such as concordance therapy, family therapy and cognitive behaviour therapy. Also consider effects on the family, carers and this man's daughter who has been witness to a range of behaviours and beliefs that she would not have the perspective to understand. Some educational, supportive and non-stigmatizing work would be essential here. When in the recovery phase, relapse prevention strategies can be planned.

Key Points

- Clozapine is indicated in the treatment of TRS.
- Clozapine treatment should be closely supervised.

CASE 60: LOW MOOD AND TIRED ALL OF THE TIME

History

A 37-year-old woman presents to her general practitioner (GP) complaining of feeling 'tired all the time'. This has come on over the last 6 months and she believes it is related to coping with three children ages 12, 7 and 5. She says that her self-esteem has been low recently and this is made worse by having no work (she was a nurse before she had children). It is also related to gradual weight gain. Her husband is supportive. She says she has found it increasingly difficult to concentrate. She has been weepy recently but has no thoughts of self-harm or harm to others. On systematic enquiry of her health, there is nothing of note except a history of constipation, which she puts down to lethargy and lack of exercise. She also has heavy periods. She is sleeping well, and sometimes feels unrefreshed by sleep. She can enjoy herself, and says she enjoys her food, and indeed has put on a few pounds recently.

Mental state examination

She is wearing a track suit and her clean hair is tied back behind her head. Her eye contact is within normal limits. She looks tired and her skin is dry. She describes her thoughts as slow and her mood as intermittently low. She is happy to chat and there is no evidence of thought disorder, thought passivity, hallucinations or delusions.

Her pulse is 62 beats per minute and her blood pressure is 140/86 mm Hg. Cardiovascular examination is otherwise unremarkable. Her skin looks dry but no other examination is performed.

Questions

- What diagnoses do you consider?
- What further examination and investigations would you carry out?

ANSWER 60

Feeling 'tired all the time' is one of the most common symptoms that a GP will see. For this reason gathering evidence of other symptoms or signs becomes crucial in narrowing down the differential diagnosis. This means enquiry into both physical and mental health problems.

Early pregnancy, stress, poor sleep and poor nutritional intake are the most common causes of tiredness. It is important to rule out more serious psychological or psychiatric problems. Depression and anxiety cause tiredness as do some somatization disorders. A range of medications and recreational drugs can also cause tiredness and this should be enquired about particularly if new medications have recently been introduced.

Infections can cause tiredness as can chronic fatigue syndrome. Ask about thirst, nocturia or polyuria to exclude diabetes or renal failure. Cardiac problems (e.g. failure, valve disease) should also be excluded. Anaemia, liver failure, coeliac disease, cancer, Parkinson disease, alcohol overuse and rare disorders such as myasthenia gravis and motor neurone disease can also cause tiredness. Endocrine causes such as Addison disease, hypopituitary, Cushing disease and hypothyroidism also need considering. This woman's symptoms should raise suspicion of hypothyroidism given the combination of fatigue, low mood, constipation, lethargy, heavy periods, weight gain and dry skin.

! Causes of hypothyroidism

- Hypothalamic failure (not producing enough Thyrotropin Releasing Hormone to stimulate the pituitary)
- Pituitary gland damage (tumour radiation or surgery)
- Autoimmune disease (Hashimoto thyroiditis is a common cause)
- Direct insult to the thyroid (radiation, surgery)
- Iodine deficiency
- Post-partum thyroiditis
- Lithium treatment

Referral to a physician is appropriate in these circumstances for further investigation, before you make any decisions about either treatment for depression or referral for mental health care. Investigations would tend to depend on the full systematic enquiry but would certainly include thyroid function tests, full blood count, blood sugar, urea and electrolytes and liver function tests in the first instance. Treatment for hypothyroidism would include thyroid replacement therapy and careful monitoring of progress including mental state.

Key Points

- There are many causes of tiredness, and a careful history should be taken to lead you towards the correct diagnosis and avoid unnecessary investigations.
- Hypothyroidism can mimic depression and vice versa.

CASE 61: A PROFOUNDLY DEAF MAN 'HEARING VOICES'

History

You are asked to see a 40-year-old man in the emergency department who is deaf. He is with a British Sign Language (BSL) interpreter who has been called in urgently by the emergency staff. The man presented with a hearing female friend who told the receptionist that she was worried about her friend, because he had been acting strangely and had told her that he was 'hearing voices'. The friend has to leave because she has to pick her children up from school, but she is still present when you arrive and he is happy for her to give some background information with him, which the interpreter signs. You discover that he has been deaf from birth, but has no other medical problems. He is single and works in a bakery on the early shift. He has a small group of friends with whom he has meals and goes to the pub. His parents who are hearing live nearby and are also supportive. He describes that for the last month he has been hearing voices. When you clarify this it transpires that what he means is that he sees images of the voice signing and lips moving, when there is no one around. He believes that they are real, and is clear that they are not his thoughts or in his mind. He does not hear any noises as such but he knows it is a male and says negative things very clearly such as 'bad man', 'devil' and 'kill yourself'. On further enquiry he reports that he has been low in mood for the last 6 weeks since a relationship with a woman he has been seeing for 9 months broke down. He had hoped they would marry, but she is now pulling back from the relationship and says that she wants to be his friend. He is concerned that he may never get married.

Mental state examination

He makes good eye contact and watches you intently. You notice that he is very expressive with his face and that his face can be contorted at times as he communicates. He is also very expressive with his hands and the movements he makes are sometimes slow and sometimes very rapid. He seems on edge. He reports being 'very sad' and seems objectively low in mood. He is tearful when discussing his ex-girlfriend. He appears to be describing hallucinatory experiences, and you are clear that these are more than thoughts. He has no delusions of persecution or paranoid ideas, although is worried about his future. He has no thought passivity experiences (thought withdrawal, insertion or broadcast) nor any delusions of control. He is orientated in time, place and person.

Questions

- What are the strange hallucinatory experiences that this man is describing?
- What treatments are likely to help this man?

ANSWER 61

Deaf people who can hear some sound, or deaf people born hearing, can experience sound in their hallucinations. Profoundly deaf people can hallucinate but they will have images of signs or lips moving, both of which are part of sign language. The language centres in the brain (Broca and Wernicke areas) are both in fully working order in deaf people who use signing (e.g. BSL). These centres are 'language' centres, not just speech centres. It is therefore not surprising that 'auditory' hallucinations are experienced in the person's first language, in the case of a deaf person, BSL.

Strong facial expressions and expressive hand movements are normal in BSL and should not be misinterpreted as signs of mental illness. Deaf awareness sessions for staff will help in understanding this better. The deaf culture is traditionally very strong with many deaf people using BSL as their preferred language and having a strong local community. This may be particularly so for deaf people born to deaf parents. Over 90% of deaf people are born to hearing parents.

Although it is important to exclude schizophrenia or organic illness leading to psychotic experiences, this man is likely to be suffering from psychotic depression and you should go through a comprehensive history with him, including depression criteria (see Case 82), and carry out an assessment of risk (Cases 33, 81 and elsewhere). Do this with a qualified interpreter.

! Definitions of levels of deafness*

Taken in testing as the better ear average over five frequencies: 0.25, 0.5, 1, 2 and 4 kilohertz (kHz).

Mild:	20–40 dB	Difficulty following speech
Moderate:	41–70 dB	Likely to need hearing aid to hear speech
Severe:	71–95 dB	Likely to rely on lip reading and hearing aid
Profound:	>95 dB	Unable to hear and understand a shouted voice Likely to be a sign language user

* British Society of Audiology. 2011. *Pure Tone Air and Bone Conduction Threshold Audiometry with and without Masking and Determination of Uncomfortable Loudness Levels.* http://www.thebsa.org.uk/wp-content/uploads/2011/04/Pure-Tone-Audiometry-1.pdf

Support for him should be culturally sensitive, and there are several adult mental health services in the country specifically for deaf people. There are also four main (and six subsidiary) centres for child and adolescent mental health. Particularly for deaf people with complex or severe problems, these centres should be utilized where possible. Where generic services are accessed it is essential to have good communication and this means arranging a qualified interpreter for any meetings. A good care plan would likely include cognitive behaviour therapy delivered in BSL, good social support from family and friends, continued employment if possible and a gradual 'back to work' plan if not, possibly a deaf support group if available, and pharmacotherapy (serotonin reuptake inhibitor and possibly atypical antipsychotic) if necessary.

Key Points

- Be deaf aware and have an understanding of deaf culture and communication needs.
- Deaf people can experience language-based hallucinations. For profoundly deaf people this is in signs and lip patterns.
- Use a qualified interpreter if you are not fluent in BSL and are communicating with a BSL user.

CASE 62: I AM SURE I AM NOT WELL

History

A single 65-year-old woman presents for her sixth visit in as many weeks. She attends with non-specific, vague concerns. She seems anxious about her physical health and requests repeated examinations and tests to be reassured that she is okay. She has a history of mild anxiety but nothing else of note. On conversation you discover that she has recently retired and a close friend of hers has died. She and the friend had intended to travel on her retirement. She now wonders whether she is in a fit state to be travelling. She has spent quite a lot of time researching illness in her age group and wants to know how she should take care of herself so she has a happy and healthy retirement. She seems particularly worried that she is likely to get cancer of the uterus as she has never had children. She is also concerned that because her parents died of heart problems in their 70s, her own risk is high.

Physical examination

She is a healthy looking slim woman. There is no evidence of any mental illness and physical examination is unremarkable.

Investigations

	Levels	*Reference range*
Haemoglobin	12.8 g/dL	11.7–15.7 g/dL
White cell count	8.8 × 10^9/L	3.5–11.0 × 10^9/L
Platelets	280 × 10^9/L	150–440 × 10^9/L
Sodium	139 mmol/L	135–145 mmol/L
Potassium	3.5 mmol/L	3.5–5.0 mmol/l
Urea	4.4 mmol/L	2.5–6.7 mmol/L
Creatinine	75 µmol/L	70–120 µmol/L
Alkaline phosphatase	88 IU/L	30–300 IU/L
Alanine aminotransferase	12 IU/L	5–35 IU/L
Gamma-glutamyl transpeptidase	32 IU/L	11–51 IU/L

Questions

- What is the likely problem?
- What advice would you give this woman?

ANSWER 62

This woman may be struggling to cope with the many changes her life has undergone. She is at risk of developing a depressive illness. Hypochondriacal disorder should be considered, but her worries are more likely to represent an adjustment disorder in the context of bereavement and retirement.

! Hypochondriacal disorder

Hypochondriacal disorder is where a person has persistent preoccupations that he or she may have physical illness or illnesses. The person reports ongoing physical symptoms (or a preoccupation about his or her physical appearance) and may worry specifically about specific organs.

It is often necessary to carry out examination and investigations as a mechanism for reassurance, but regular and repeated tests may lead to heightening of anxiety as they can reinforce ruminations about health.

To minimize the likelihood of developing problems she should be advised to

- Schedule regular social activities so she does not become socially isolated.
- Ensure that she continues to take good care of herself by eating well and exercising regularly.
- Consider some voluntary activities, as being mentally and physically engaged helps with both physical but especially mental health. It can also help to keep things in perspective.
- Learn a new skill or do something she may not have had time to do before.
- Join social groups, which means that she has events to look forward to.
- Get advice from groups targeted at older people to help adjust to her new life stage.

Key Points

- Regular attendance with non-specific concerns may be a presentation of depressive illness or anxiety disorder.
- Constant reassurance and repeated tests may prove to be unhelpful strategies.

CASE 63: REPEATING THE SAME STORY OVER AND OVER AGAIN

History

A 76-year-old retired surveyor is brought to surgery by his wife. She reports that he has gradually stopped reading and writing, both activities he used to enjoy. He has a tendency to repeat things many times during the day, apparently unaware that he has mentioned them earlier. He also has more difficulty putting sentences together, and forgets the names of common objects such as the radiator and the radio. He has become slightly more clumsy. He recently failed to recognize a cousin whom he had not seen for a year. He tells the doctor that he is fine and that his wife is making a fuss about nothing. The previous week he wanted to return a form to claim a chance to win a large prize from a mailshot designed to encourage him to attend a promotional Spanish Apartment Share meeting. He would previously have recognized this as a promotion and put it straight in the bin. He drinks a small bottle of beer twice a week, usually at the weekends, and is a non-smoker. He has not been lethargic or disinhibited and continues to get great pleasure from gardening. His wife describes that onset has been gradual, so much so that she was prompted to take action by their daughter.

Mental state examination

Mental state examination shows that he has good eye contact and sits still in a chair throughout the interview. His speech is slightly laboured and on several occasions he seems to struggle to find the right word. None of his sentences are long or complex. He has no pressure of speech or flight of ideas. Occasionally he will lose the thread of what he is saying and stop talking or start on a different topic. He is uncertain why he is being interviewed. There is no psychomotor retardation or agitation. There is no evidence of hallucinations or psychosis, although his wife says that he sometimes wakes up in the middle of the night thinking that there is an intruder in the bedroom. His Mini Mental State Examination score is 19. He thinks he is in the general practitioner (GP) surgery when in fact he is at the local hospital.

Physical examination is unremarkable, including neurological examination, and he is well nourished. He has some mild eczema. He has good peripheral pulses, no carotid bruits and a blood pressure of 115/70 mm Hg.

> **! Mini Mental State Examination**
>
> The Mini Mental State Examination (MMSE) is a 30-item questionnaire introduced by Folstein, Folstein and McHugh (1975) that tests for orientation in time and place, attention, registration, recall, arithmetic skills, expressive and receptive language and motor skills. A score of less than 27 may suggest some cognitive impairment. A score below 20 may be described as reflecting moderate impairment and below 10 severe.
>
> * Folstein MF, Folstein SE, McHugh PR. 1975. Mini-mental state: A practical method for grading the cognitive state of patients for the clinician. *Journal of Psychiatric Research* 12, 189–198.

Questions

- What is the differential diagnosis?
- What further questions would you need to ask?
- What advice can you give the couple about treatment?

ANSWER 63

Differential diagnosis

Alzheimer dementia is the most likely cause. There is no evidence of Parkinson disease or Huntington disease on examination, and Creutzfeldt–Jakob disease is unlikely given the history. The absence of lethargy or disinhibition makes frontotemporal dementia unlikely. It will be important to exclude depression by further history and discussion with his wife. Dementia with Lewy bodies usually involves parkinsonian features (although these may not be evident early in the illness) and often involves visual hallucinations, alongside attentional problems, fluctuating abilities and planning (executive functioning) difficulties. Cortico-basal ganglionic degeneration also involves parkinsonism and signs of cortical atrophy including dyspraxia, dysphasia, cortical sensory loss and action tremor. Progressive supranuclear palsy would usually involve regular falls, slow blinking, dry eyes, tunnel vision, slurred speech and swallowing problems followed by further movement problems including walking difficulties. Vascular dementia is typically described as progressing with step-wise deterioration. It is more likely in the presence of a history of hypertension, diabetes, vascular disease or smoking.

What further questions would you need to ask?

It is important to exclude depression, since this would lead to an alternative set of treatments. Some of the symptoms presenting here are also typical of depression in the elderly such as reduced ability to concentrate (e.g. on reading), reduced energy and apparent memory loss. Ask about inability to enjoy oneself (anhedonia), weepiness, irritability, feelings of guilt or worthlessness, anxiety and effects on sleep or appetite. Also ask about whether life is worth living. It is important to check sensitively for suicidal thoughts and plans in depression. An assessment of dementia should also include enquiry into functioning in all activities of daily living, and an assessment of risk in all domains (including driving).

Advice about treatment

Cholinesterase inhibitors such as donepezil, rivastigmine and galantamine are not a cure but can slow the progression of dementia, reduce apathy and improve alertness and mood in Alzheimer disease and are approved (National Institute for Health and Care Excellence [NICE]) for the management of mild and moderate Alzheimer disease. Memantine, the extrasynaptic blocker of the *N*-methyl-D-aspartate (NMDA) subtype of glutamate receptors (NMDAR), is approved for the management of severe Alzheimer disease and where cholinesterase inhibitors cannot be used. They can also improve everyday task performance. Antipsychotics are sometimes used to treat severe behavioural and psychological symptoms in dementia (such as aggression or agitation), but their use is not without risk so should only be considered if the symptoms are associated with psychosis and the symptoms are severe. They are not appropriate here.

The assessment should inform the creation of a care package where the patient's circumstances indicate that one is required. Carer support is an essential component of the management of dementia, so offer contact information for sources of support such as the Alzheimer's Society. As dementia progresses social services and mental health services work together to shape a care plan with the family. Setting up lasting power of attorney arrangements early can avoid unnecessary financial and legal complications later on.

As the illness progresses environmental alterations such as use of clocks, calendars, lists and physical support such as rails will help. A comprehensive multidisciplinary team will include occupational therapists, physiotherapists, psychologists and social workers as well as community psychiatric nurses and psychiatrists. Advice to establish a routine with activities, stimulation and conversation all give traction to life, and may maintain mood. Therapy geared to improving reality orientation, with regular stimulation, has been shown to help. With further progression of the illness, the patient's care needs will change and, although the goal should be to support the patient in his or her own environment as long as this is safe and sensible, the time may come when a move into more supported accommodation or 24-hour care becomes appropriate.

Key Points

- Early detection of dementia allows support and interventions to be planned.
- It is important to rule out depression.
- Cholinesterase inhibitors are currently recommended by NICE for people with moderate Alzheimer disease (MMSE score of 10–20).

CASE 64: INCREASINGLY FORGETFUL, CONFUSED AND SUSPICIOUS

History

A 66-year-old bank manager is brought to the emergency department by his wife and his daughter, as he has had a flurry of 'blank episodes'. He became unresponsive for a minute or so and appeared confused for 2–3 minutes. He then reverted to his normal state with little memory of what had happened. The final episode has left him with a drooping face, which has now recovered. However, he seems to have word-finding difficulty. He took early retirement 18 months ago after he developed slurred speech and confusion in a similar episode. Following that episode, he recovered quite well but found it difficult to concentrate at work. He had a similar episode 6 months ago following which he began losing his way while driving. He has avoided driving over the past few weeks. He has become increasingly forgetful and suspicious of late. His moods are variable and he gets 'worked up' quite easily. He was helping a charity with their accounts but has been asked to leave as he made several simple errors and reacted in anger when confronted with his errors. He lives with his wife, who is very supportive. He has no previous psychiatric history but has suffered from hypertension for 20 years and diabetes type 2 for 15 years treated adequately with enalapril and metformin, respectively. He has smoked 30 cigarettes a day for 50 years. He drinks socially and does not take any illicit drugs.

Physical examination

He appears as an overweight, well-dressed gentleman who walks with a slow shuffling gait. His pulse rate is 86 beats per minute, regular, and blood pressure is 176/92 mm Hg. Central nervous system examination reveals bilateral increased tone though strength and reflexes are equal all over. There is no other physical finding of note. Funduscopic examination is normal.

Mental state examination

His eye contact is good. He is pleasant, cooperative but a little perplexed. His speech is slow and hesitant. There is evidence of psychomotor retardation and his mood is low and anxious. There is no evidence of formal thought disorder, but he does have some ideas of reference and persecution. There is evidence of cognitive impairment – he scored 21/30 on Mini Mental State Examination (MMSE) losing points on attention, recall, naming and construction. He seems to have a reasonable degree of insight and wants help to get better.

Questions

- What is the likely diagnosis?
- How will you differentiate it from Alzheimer disease?

ANSWER 64

This man is presenting with an abrupt onset of word-finding difficulty, which is occurring in the context of transient neurological signs with no residual deficit. He has an increased risk of cardiovascular disease with history of hypertension, diabetes mellitus and smoking. He has experienced a transient ischaemic attack, which resolves completely in less than 24 hours and often much more quickly. He has had similar episodes each of which has been followed by further cognitive deterioration. Impaired daily functioning and evidence of cognitive impairments in multiple domains are suggestive of dementia. Abrupt, step-wise cognitive impairment with a cardiovascular risk history is very suggestive of multi-infarct or vascular dementia (VD), which is the second most common cause of dementia after Alzheimer disease (AD). AD has a chronic, insidious course with an equal male:female ratio, whereas males are more at risk of VD. Hachinski Ischemic Score (see Table 64.1) may be useful in attempting to differentiate between the two conditions though, in practice, 20%–30% of cases may have both AD and VD. Making the right diagnosis has treatment implications, as acetylcholinesterase inhibitors are indicated for the treatment of cognitive and non-cognitive symptoms of AD but are not licensed for the treatment of VD. Atypical antipsychotics are associated with increased relative risk of stroke in patients with vascular dementia, so they should only be used after careful consideration (and discussion with the patient and/or their carers) of the risks and potential benefits.

Table 64.1 **Hachinski ischaemic scale**

Clinical feature	Score
Abrupt onset	2
Step-wise deterioration	1
Fluctuating course	1
Nocturnal confusion	1
Relative preservation of personality	1
Depression	1
Somatic complaints	1
Emotional incontinence	1
History of hypertension	1
History of strokes	2
Evidence of associated atherosclerosis	1
Focal neurological symptoms	2
Focal neurological signs	2

Note: A score of greater than 7 is suggestive of multi-infarct dementia while less than 4 is suggestive of Alzheimer disease.

Radiological evidence of cerebrovascular pathology (on computed tomography or magnetic resonance imaging) can lend support to a diagnosis of VD.

Key Points

- Step-wise cognitive deterioration with a cardiovascular risk history is suggestive of multi-infarct dementia.
- Psychiatric symptoms such as depression and anxiety may be prominent.

CASE 65: SEEING FLIES ON THE CEILING

History

You visit a 67-year-old man at home who is reported as being confused. His wife is distressed because he repeatedly asks her to swat the flies from the ceiling, when she can see nothing there. He has been in bed for 3 days with a 'cold'. He frequently gets up and wanders around without knowing where he is going. His wife says on one occasion he burst out laughing without any reason that she could discern. At other times he seems bewildered. She describes that he becomes more confused in the evening and at night, and has urinated in the cupboard. He has no diarrhoea. A week ago he was well and able to do gardening. He has not been confused until recently. On questioning his wife says that while he occasionally forgets the names of village acquaintances, his memory has otherwise been fine. He is not a large user of alcohol and drinks only a small bottle of beer or a sherry once per week. His wife has remained well throughout.

Mental state examination

When you visit he is lying in bed. He is initially suspicious of you and asks if you are an undertaker. He is preoccupied with stripes on the wallpaper and asks his wife several times to get some towels to mop up the water running down the wall. He makes poor eye contact. He is slightly restless in bed and looks dishevelled. There is a strong body odour. He looks perplexed and frightened. He does not appear to be responding to voices, and his wife says he has not mentioned this. He is not able to answer questions about passivity experiences. With respect to delusions his wife says that he thought that she was going to stab him when she was trying to spoon-feed him some soup the previous night. He pushed her away but has not hit her. He is unable to say what day of the week it is or what time of day. He names the previous prime minister as the current one, and cannot repeat back an address that you give him to remember. He thinks he is in hospital. You need to repeat questions as he seems preoccupied with his own thoughts or things that he is seeing.

Physical examination

There are no abdominal signs and the cardiovascular system seems normal with good peripheral pulses. His heart rate is 96 beats per minute and his blood pressure is 110/68 mm Hg. His temperature is normal. He has poor air entry and crackles over the right side of the lower lung, and he has bronchial breathing and dulled percussion in the same area. He has an increased respiratory rate.

Questions

- What is the most likely diagnosis and what are the possible causes?
- What is the management at this point?

ANSWER 65

He is disorientated in time and place and has clouding of consciousness. It is likely that he has delirium. This can be caused by anything that disturbs the functioning of the brain. This usually involves interference with the metabolism, perfusion or oxygenation of the brain. More specifically it will be important to rule out malnutrition, dehydration, drug intoxication or withdrawal states, poisoning, infections (urinary tract infection, septicaemia, chest infection, etc.), sleep deprivation and head injury. Sometimes it may occur post surgery and could be related to a range of possible factors including deoxygenation, brain injury, infection or unbalanced metabolism.

The history suggests little evidence of gradual dementia, although vascular dementia may progress with step-wise deteriorations.

Treatment involves two main aspects. The first is to treat the underlying cause. This needs careful assessment to make sure that nothing is missed. The second is to treat the distress or discomfort symptomatically. Sedatives or major tranquilizers for the latter are only used when absolutely necessary and when the underlying cause has been identified. Doses should be reviewed every 24 hours. Haloperidol (or lorazepam for patients with Lewy body dementia or Parkinson disease) is commonly used. Some use risperidone as an alternative.

The lung signs in this situation suggest pneumonia and the absence of a fever does not exclude this as a cause. The mainstay of treatment is directed at the cause. Consider treating the infection with antibiotics, ensuring adequate hydration and nutrition, identifying metabolic disturbance and providing corrective treatments, ensuring adequate oxygenation, and identifying any poisoning or withdrawal states and providing necessary treatments.

Poisoning seems unlikely since his wife is well, but doctors should remain vigilant to causes such as carbon monoxide poisoning in these situations. He has not had diarrhoea but may have a urinary tract infection. He has had a cold so an undiagnosed pneumonia is possible. Drug or alcohol states seem unlikely given the history as does head injury although he may have knocked his head without his wife knowing.

Rather than organizing tests and waiting for the results a hospital admission is appropriate to investigate and provide necessary treatment.

Key Points

- Delirium affects attention, consciousness, perception, thinking, memory and emotions.
- There are usually behavioural effects and an impact on the sleep–wake cycle.

CASE 66: COGNITIVE IMPAIRMENT WITH VISUAL HALLUCINATIONS

History

A 78-year-old man attends the general practitioner (GP) surgery with his daughter for an urgent appointment as his eyes have been rolling upwards uncontrollably since this morning. He lives on his own following the death of his wife last year and has been very low since then. His daughter is very concerned about him. His self-care has suffered and he often burns his food though at other times 'he seems completely fine'. Three months ago, he suffered a fall and bruised his face. His daughter has noticed other bruises on his body. He has developed a tremor and seems to stumble a lot. His sleep and appetite have been poor and he has lost about 2 kg in weight over the past year. Two days ago, he went to the GP surgery complaining of seeing a whole orchestra playing in his kitchen and was prescribed haloperidol 0.5 mg twice daily. However, since yesterday, he has been suffering uncontrollable twisting movement of his neck and face. Last night, he could not keep his balance and suffered a fall in his lounge.

Mental state examination

He is pleasant but seems a little confused and bewildered. He does not have any formal thought disorder. He describes in great detail the musicians in the orchestra that he can see in his kitchen. He acknowledges that they are not real and says he finds them disconcerting but not particularly unpleasant. His mood is low and he gets tearful during the interview. Abbreviated Mental Test is abnormal with a score of 5 out of 10. He has reasonable insight into his symptoms and wants treatment to get better. Physical examination reveals a resting tremor in his hands with cogwheel rigidity in his forearms. The rest of the physical examination is unremarkable.

! Abbreviated Mental Test

1. What is your age (within 1 year)?
2. What is the time to the nearest hour?
3. What is the year?
4. What is the name of this place?

Give the patient an address (e.g. 42 West St, Leeds), and ask him or her to repeat it at the end of the test.

1. What is your birthday (date and month)?
2. In what year did the First World War begin?
3. What is the King or Queen's name?
4. Can you recognize…? (Can the patient identify two people around him or her?)
5. Please count from 20 backwards to 1.
6. Can you remember the address which I gave you?

* Hodkinson HM. 1972. Evaluation of a mental test score for assessment of mental impairment in the elderly. *Age and Ageing* 1, 233–238.

Questions

- What is the differential diagnosis?
- What is the pharmacological management?

ANSWER 66

This man is presenting with cognitive impairment, neuroleptic medication-induced dystonia (upward rolling of eyes), extrapyramidal rigidity and tremor, vivid hallucinations, repeated falls and fluctuating consciousness. This combination of symptoms is strongly suggestive of dementia with Lewy bodies (DLB). DLB is one of the most common causes of dementia after Alzheimer disease (AD). Misdiagnosis is common because of its unusual presentation: often with psychiatric symptoms such as visual hallucinations and depression rather than memory impairment. Falls are an early feature as are parkinsonian symptoms.

! Differential diagnosis

- Alzheimer dementia: insidious and chronic progressive cognitive impairment without fluctuations. Hallucinations are usually not prominent and parkinsonian symptoms are seen late in the illness.
- Vascular dementia: step-wise deterioration with history of cardiovascular risk factors is seen.
- Other causes of dementia: such as fronto-temporal dementia (behavioural disinhibition), prion diseases (rapidly progressive, characteristic periodic complexes on electroencephalogram) and progressive supranuclear palsy (insidious onset with vertical gaze palsy).
- Psychotic disorder: schizophrenia may mimic DLB due to visual hallucinations and delusions but falls, cognitive impairment and neuroleptic sensitivity are usually absent.
- Depression: may often be a presenting symptom of DLB. Low mood, sleep and appetite disturbance and cognitive changes may all point to depression but the characteristic features of DLB such as falls, extrapyramidal rigidity and neuroleptic sensitivity are absent.

Magnetic resonance imaging (MRI) scan is essential to rule out vascular dementia and other brain pathology. Single photon emission computed tomography (SPECT) scan with a specific ligand can confirm the loss of dopaminergic neurons in DLB while there are no such changes seen in AD. There is no specific cure. Acetylcholinesterase inhibitors may be helpful for treatment of non-cognitive symptoms such as delusions, hallucinations and challenging behaviour. If acetylcholinesterase inhibitors are ineffective, typical antipsychotics such as haloperidol should be avoided. Instead atypical antipsychotics such as quetiapine or aripiprazole may be helpful but vigilance for extra-pyramidal side effects is still essential. Depression, when present, should be treated with selective serotonin reuptake inhibitors such as citalopram or fluoxetine. A care package with carer support and a full range of psychosocial interventions should be put into place.

Key Points

- Fluctuating consciousness, visual hallucinations, history of falls and parkinsonian symptoms suggest a diagnosis of DLB.
- Acetylcholinesterase inhibitors are first-line and atypical antipsychotics second-line treatments for distressing non-cognitive symptoms.

CASE 67: I THINK MY WIFE IS POISONING MY FOOD

History

A 79-year-old man presents with his family. They are concerned that his behaviour has become more unpredictable. He has also started to become more and more suspicious of all his family members, particularly his wife. He thinks she is poisoning him and will now no longer eat anything she has cooked. He does not even trust her to make him a drink. He has become more hostile and aggressive, which is a big change as he has always been a quiet-spoken and gentle man. His sleep is disturbed and his appetite has increased with some weight gain. He has no past psychiatric history.

He has a complex medical history and his family report that he has most recently been treated for pulmonary fibrosis which had been relatively stable. However, following a bout of pneumonia his breathing was compromised so a new regime of medication was started. He is on 5 mg prednisolone three times daily and has been taking this for 6 weeks. The family report he had a course of steroids previously but did not have any side effects from it so they do not think it is causing problems.

Mental state examination

The patient is overweight and slightly breathless. He is clearly suspicious of his family watching and listening carefully. He does not hear well and you often have to repeat your questions. When you turn away to answer a question from his son, he immediately assumes that you and the family are plotting against him. His speech is fast but clear. His mood is difficult to assess as at times he seems fine but then will become quickly irritated. He admits he has had some auditory hallucinations which are somewhat unclear. The voices tell him to be careful of his wife as she is trying to kill him. He is convinced his children have started visiting more because they are in cahoots with his wife. He is also convinced that he could look after himself without any help from his family. He has not had any self-harm ideation or plans.

He is orientated in time, place and person. His short-term memory is poor and he is easily frustrated when he becomes aware that he has got something wrong. He is not really aware of recent world or national events despite saying he reads the paper daily. He also admits that because he was more breathless he had increased his doses of prednisolone.

Questions

- What is the likely diagnosis?
- How would you manage the psychosis?
- How would you explain the psychosis to the family?

ANSWER 67

The most likely diagnosis is side effects of his prednisolone medication. However differential diagnosis would need to exclude organic psychosis, dementia, depression and bipolar disorder.

The most immediate plan of action would be to reduce the steroids as it is most likely that they have caused this problem. Steroids cause a number of side effects including changes in mental health. Mild mental changes are occasionally observed after a few days of treatment and may include excitation, euphoria, hypomania and insomnia. Patients initially on high steroid doses may become manic, excitable and incur personality changes. They may appear extremely cheerful, be talkative, have boundless energy, make impulsive decisions and feel the need for significantly less rest or sleep. This can cause strain on relationships with carers and loved ones. However paranoid psychosis is also not uncommon.

It may also be useful to get his hearing tested as hearing impairment may make his paranoid thoughts and feelings worse.

The family needs to have the mental health side effects of steroids explained to them. They also need to be told how to watch for early changes so that they can pre-empt problems in the future. Given his medical condition it may not be possible to completely stop the steroids, but a mechanism should be put into place with the family for ensuring he takes the correct dosage and that his response to it is monitored.

! Paranoia

Paranoia can occur in many contexts. It may be part of a personality disorder with a long-standing mistrust about other people. If it is delusional in intensity it may be part of a psychotic disorder such as persistent delusional disorder or schizophrenia or part of a manic–depressive or depressive psychosis. It could also be part of a transient or drug-induced psychotic disorder.

Key Points

- In the elderly, even small doses of steroids can cause significant mental health side effects.
- The elderly are often on several different medications so care needs to be taken as interactions are highly likely.

CASE 68: ACUTE AGITATION IN A MEDICAL INPATIENT

History

A 72-year-old man is admitted to try to achieve better control of his diabetes which has to date been controlled using diet. There is no other medical history of note. He had a short depressive illness in his 40s following the death of his mother. He had settled well onto the ward but after his wife left he became increasingly agitated and restless.

Mental state examination

The man is cooperative and communicative but clearly very distressed and easily distracted. He is somewhat shaky. His speech is normal and he describes himself as worried but cannot say what is worrying him. There is no evidence of any psychosis.

He is orientated in time, place and person. He is able to repeat back the names of three objects that you identify for him. He is able to spell WORLD backwards though requires two attempts. He is also able to do the serial sevens test but falters after four subtractions. He is able to recall the three objects identified earlier in the examination. There is nothing to suggest that he does not understand what is said to him.

Physical examination

The man is rather obese. His pupils are dilated and he is sweating but is apyrexial. His blood pressure is 135/85 mm Hg.

Investigations

	Levels	*Reference range*
Haemoglobin	14.4 g/dL	13.3–17.7 g/dL
Mean corpuscular volume (MCV)	85 fL	80–99 fL
White cell count	8.8×10^9/L	$3.9–11.0 \times 10^9$/L
Platelets	280×10^9/L	$150–440 \times 10^9$/L
Sodium	139 mmol/L	135–145 mmol/L
Potassium	3.5 mmol/L	3.5–5.0 mmol/l
Urea	2.9 mmol/L	2.5–6.7 mmol/L
Creatinine	75 µmol/L	70–120 µmol/L
Blood glucose	3 mmol/L	4–8 mmol/L
Alkaline phosphatase	151 IU/L	30–300 IU/L
Alanine aminotransferase	26 IU/L	5–35 IU/L
Gamma-glutamyl transpeptidase	35 IU/L	11–51 IU/L
Bilirubin	12 mmol/L	3–17 mmol/L

Questions

- What is the likely cause of this man's agitation?
- How should he be managed?
- What are the psychiatric causes of agitation?
- What medications are effective in managing agitation?

ANSWER 68

The first task is to identify what his agitation is related to. If he is agitated because of an underlying medical issue, that needs to be addressed first. Medical causes include hyper- or hypoglycaemia (as here), electrolyte disturbance, renal or hepatic failure, thyroid or adrenal disorders, Wernicke encephalopathy, hypotension, heart failure, neurological disorders (e.g. stroke), infection of all kinds (especially in the elderly), including meningitis, and dementia. Agitation can also be caused by hunger, constipation, pain and sleep deprivation. It will also be necessary to look carefully at his medication as steroids, anticholinergics, barbiturates, amphetamines and antipsychotics may all cause agitation.

If no medical cause is found, then you need to explore psychiatric causes. Underlying psychiatric disorders such as anxiety or psychosis with delusional thinking need to be treated with the relevant medication. Depression is commonly missed in the elderly. It is also important to be aware of substance (especially alcohol) problems in the elderly as the pattern may relate more to a regular controlled drinker than someone who binges. Abuse of or dependence on medically prescribed medication which may be stopped at the time of admission may also cause agitation. Recent stressful life events may also lead to agitation.

Agitation may be managed by careful nursing but it is most likely that medication will be required. If safe to do so, oral medication should be considered first. This may help the patient restore some feeling of control and ease escalating agitation.

The goals of medication in the management of acute agitation are to quickly calm the patient without excessive sedation and to ensure patient safety (and sometimes staff safety if the patient is violent with his or her agitation). However, there is also a need to nurse the patient appropriately so minimal medication is used. Lorazepam is preferred for undifferentiated agitation (provides muscle relaxation, anxiolytic, anticonvulsant effects and generalized sedation). Haloperidol has a relatively low propensity for sedation and hypotension compared with other intramuscular (IM) agents; however it is more likely to cause extrapyramidal side effects. The combination of a benzodiazepine and a typical antipsychotic (i.e. haloperidol) has been shown to be superior to monotherapy with either agent, and may allow for decreased doses of the antipsychotic medication. The combination can cause excessive sedation. After treatment with IM agents, monitor vitals and clinical status at regular intervals. Allow adequate time for clinical response between doses.

If the initial treatment fails to produce an adequate response after 2–4 hours options include the following. Give another dose of the same medication if partially effective, or a different medication if the first medication is ineffective. Give a dose of lorazepam if the first medication was an antipsychotic. Give a combination of the same antipsychotic and lorazepam (except olanzapine which needs to be given after an hour's interval). Lower starting and maximum doses need to be observed in the elderly.

Key Points

- Agitation is extremely common in elderly patients.
- Medication is very useful but needs to be used in conjunction with sensitive nursing.
- Lorazepam and/or haloperidol are probably most effective.

CASE 69: SHE IS NOT EATING OR DRINKING ANYTHING

History

A 73-year-old woman presents with a 6-month history of low mood. She had been previously relatively well and there were no major life events prior to her low mood. She had complained of being unable to sleep, unable to motivate herself to get out and about, and felt there was little hope things would ever be different. She had lost about 15 kg in weight in that period, with the last 10 kg having been lost in the last few weeks. She had been tried on fluoxetine but it had little effect. Over the last month she has developed features of psychosis with derogatory auditory hallucinations and delusions of worthlessness. She feels she should be left alone to die as she is not worth saving and other people are more deserving of the resources. She has denied any self-harm ideation but admits that she can see little point in being alive. Her food intake has gradually diminished and over the last few days she has barely eaten or drunk anything. When she was admitted she was very withdrawn and mute. No one was able to communicate with her.

Mental state examination

The woman does not respond to any questions. She does not make any eye contact. She is mute and her speech cannot be assessed. She will occasionally grunt if efforts are made to move her. She does not seem orientated in place, time or person.

Physical examination

The woman has clearly neglected self-care. She looks emaciated. Her eyes are partially closed and she does not respond to any requests. She shows marked bradykinesia (slow movement) and there is hardly any spontaneous movement. She is clinically very dehydrated.

Questions

- What is the likely diagnosis?
- What would be the most appropriate intervention?
- How would you prepare a patient for electroconvulsive therapy (ECT)?

ANSWER 69

The most likely diagnosis is depression with psychosis but you should exclude schizophrenia and any medical disorder. Because of her catatonic state ECT is likely to be an appropriate intervention after she is rehydrated and made medically safe. ECT is primarily used to treat major depressive symptoms where other treatments have been unsuccessful or where life is at risk (because of either extreme self-neglect or very high risk of suicide) when a rapid response is required. ECT involves passing a controlled dose of electricity through the brain between two electrodes applied to the head to induce an epileptiform seizure. The goal of treatment is to produce a seizure lasting 20–50 seconds. The treatment is given under a short-acting general anaesthetic, using a muscle relaxant to modify the seizure. As a general anaesthetic is required to be able to administer ECT the treatment can only be given in places where this is safely possible. Treatments are usually given twice a week, and a typical course of ECT consists of about six to ten treatments. Consent is usually obtained for a series of treatments but consent can of course be withdrawn at any point.

It is important that the patient's consent is sought prior to the treatment. There are a number of contexts in which ECT may be given. The patient might have capacity to consent to ECT and agree to treatment. The patient might lack capacity to consent but not object to treatment, in which case treatment can be given under the provisions of Section 5 of the Mental Capacity Act. The patient might lack capacity to consent and actively refuse treatment, in which case the patient may be detained under the Mental Health Act and be treated, after a second opinion has been obtained, under the provisions of Section 58 of that act. A patient detained under the Mental Health Act may require ECT as an emergency in which case treatment may be given under the provisions of Section 62 before a second opinion has been obtained. Emergency treatment is permitted to save the patient's life, prevent serious deterioration, alleviate serious suffering or prevent danger to the patient or others arising from the patient's behaviour. Prior to ECT patients will need a thorough physical examination and appropriate investigations as fitness for anaesthetic will need to be assessed.

! Side effects of ECT

The following side effects need to be explained to the patient and/or the patient's carers:

1. Transient headache, muscle soreness, nausea or agitation
2. Transient memory impairment for the period immediately before and after ECT
3. Transient confusion immediately after treatment, especially in the elderly
4. Possibility of permanent memory dysfunction or loss (although there is controversy about whether this is a result of the ECT or other factors including the depression itself)
5. Risks associated with general anaesthesia

As for any other procedure where an anaesthetic is required the patient must not have eaten or drunk anything for at least 8 hours before the treatment. Patients having outpatient ECT should not drive or operate machinery on the day of treatment and patients will normally be observed for at least 4 hours post-ECT, as is usual for any day procedure. Immediate post-anaesthetic care should be provided in an appropriately equipped recovery area by appropriately trained staff.

Key Points

- ECT is not usually a first-line treatment but remains a vital option for some patients, particularly where the life of the individual concerned is threatened and/or other treatments are ineffective.
- All the usual precautions must be taken as for any procedure involving anaesthesia.

CASE 70: A RESTLESS POSTOPERATIVE PATIENT WHO WON'T STAY IN BED

History

The nurses in the intensive care unit contact you regarding a 70-year-old postoperative male who had a hip replacement 24 hours previously. The man is extremely agitated and keeps wanting to pull out his intravenous line and get out of bed. He is quite fragile and there is real concern that he may get physically hurt if he is not restrained. He is demanding to be allowed to leave and go home. The nurses want to know whose responsibility it is to 'section' him to ensure that he can be treated.

Mental state examination

The man is uncooperative and does not answer questions. He just repeats his demands to be allowed to leave. His speech is loud and repetitive. There is no evidence of psychosis. The man cannot tell you the year, season, date, day or month. He can tell you he is in hospital but cannot understand why. He cannot register any information and immediately forgets why he cannot go home even when this is explained to him.

Physical examination

The man is clearly agitated and hostile when he is spoken to. He is connected to an IV drip and looks well hydrated. He is apyrexial. There is a bandage on his right leg with a drain. There does not seem to be any excessive bleeding. The man denies being in any pain.

Investigations

	Levels	*Reference range*
Haemoglobin	14.4 g/dL	13.3–17.7 g/dL
Mean corpuscular volume (MCV)	85 fL	80–99 fL
White cell count	8.8×10^9/L	$3.9–11.0 \times 10^9$/L
Platelets	280×10^9/L	$150–440 \times 10^9$/L
Sodium	139 mmol/L	135–145 mmol/L
Potassium	3.5 mmol/L	3.5–5.0 mmol/l
Urea	2.9 mmol/L	2.5–6.7 mmol/L
Creatinine	75 μmol/L	70–120 μmol/L
Blood glucose	6 mmol/L	4–6 mmol/L
Alkaline phosphatase	151 IU/L	30–300 IU/L
Alanine aminotransferase	26 IU/L	5–35 IU/L
Gamma-glutamyl transpeptidase	35 IU/L	11–51 IU/L
Bilirubin	12 μmol/L	3–17 μmol/L

Questions

- What is the likely diagnosis?
- How should this situation be managed?
- Under what legal frameworks can he be kept in hospital and treated against his wishes?

ANSWER 70

Some degree of postoperative delirium occurs in around 25% of elderly patients within a week of surgery. It is a transient mental dysfunction that can result in increased morbidity, delayed functional recovery and prolonged hospital stay. The distinguishing features are impaired cognition, fluctuating levels of consciousness and altered psychomotor activity. It is usually seen within a couple of days post-operation and is often worse at night. It may go unnoticed or be misdiagnosed. Patients are usually incoherent, disorientated and have impairment of memory and attention. It ranges from mild confusion to full hallucinations. As in this scenario, patients with delirium may remove vital drains or temporary pacemaker wires, or they may fall and injure themselves when getting out of bed, and so need careful monitoring.

The Mini Mental State Exam (MMSE) is useful to monitor fluctuating cognitive functioning.

Preoperative risk factors include previous history of delirium, pre-existing dementia, age over 70 years, depression, polypharmacy and drug interaction, alcohol or sedative–hypnotic withdrawal, endocrine and metabolic problems. Peri-operative hypoxia, hypocarbia and sepsis are also risk factors as are certain anaesthetics, pethidine and anticholinergics. The risk of postoperative delirium is similar with general and regional anaesthetic techniques. Regional anaesthesia may involve the use of drugs that increase the risk. Pre-existing sensory or perceptual deficits, fluid and electrolyte imbalance, sleep deprivation (e.g. from a busy ward) and an inability to keep track of time can all contribute to confusion and disorientation.

! Nursing patients with delirium

- Give regular reassurance and reorientation.
- Use clear communication.
- Minimize noise and have adequate lighting (but not too bright).
- Use relaxation strategies such as music, etc. Avoid unnecessary waking.
- Encourage familiar family or friends to stay.
- Keep consistent carers and avoid regular moves.
- Avoid restraint and use strategies to maintain oxygenation and mobility.
- Avoid invasive interventions if possible.
- Use medication only as a last resort.

The underlying organic cause of the delirium should be found and treated. If medication is necessary, antipsychotics (e.g. haloperidol or the newer, atypical antipsychotics) are generally preferable to benzodiazepines. For acute control of delirium, oral haloperidol at a dose of 0.5 mg with a minimum interval of 2 hours is the preferred treatment. For more agitated patients, intramuscular haloperidol can be used. The maximum total dose in 24 hours should not usually exceed 5 mg. For patients with Parkinson disease or Lewy body dementia an appropriate alternative is lorazepam 0.5–1 mg orally up to a maximum dose of 3 mg in 24 hours with a minimum interval of 2 hours between doses.

After recovery from an acute episode, a psychiatric or psychosocial assessment may aid early functional rehabilitation.

Section 5 of the Mental Capacity Act is the legal framework under which treatment can be given to a patient who lacks capacity to consent to that treatment. The treatment must be necessary and in that person's best interests. In this case the patient's inability to retain the information necessary to make an informed decision about his care demonstrates lack of capacity. This should be carefully documented. This capacity assessment can be carried out by the treating surgeons. Restraint of a patient who lacks capacity is only allowed to prevent harm and provided that the restraint is proportionate to both the likelihood and the seriousness of that harm. Keeping this patient in hospital against his will to treat delirium will prevent him from suffering serious harm.

The Mental Health Act can only be used to assess or treat mental disorder. Although delirium can be construed as a mental disorder, and treatment of the underlying physical cause of the delirium can be considered treatment for the mental disorder of delirium, the Mental Capacity Act provides a much clearer framework for the delivery of care against a patient's wishes under these circumstances.

Key Points

- Postoperative delirium is common in the elderly.
- Nursing care is key.

CASE 71: MOOD CHANGES

History

A 71-year-old ex-cleaner is brought to the follow-up neurology clinic by her daughter and a carer from the residential home where she resides. She has been diagnosed with Parkinson disease for 7 years and has managed reasonably well with a combination tablet of carbidopa 25 mg and levodopa 200 mg, two tablets four times daily. Her cognition has been worsening gradually from a Mini Mental State Examination score of 24/30 about 2 years ago to 20/30 on her current visit. She reports no change in herself but her daughter says that over the past 6 months her mother has been exhibiting periods of 'weird behaviour' – screaming and shouting for hours followed by periods of tearfulness and uncontrollable sobbing. When agitated, she has been disinhibited, taking her clothes off and swearing in a manner very uncharacteristic of her. She sings loudly and cheerfully making everyone laugh with 'lewd jokes'. When tearful, she has appeared profoundly slowed down and has spoken of wanting to stay in bed, not being able to face the day ahead. Her sleep has been disturbed and so has her appetite. At times, she has refused to go down to the dining room. Her mobility has worsened. Her shuffling gait and tremors have worsened and so too her bradykinesia. According to her carer, her personality has changed a lot over the past year or so. She has become more reserved and does not enjoy bingo or shopping trips. She does look forward to her daughter's visits, but of late has not been as enthusiastic as she used to be. Her daughter visits her three times a week and is very close to her. Her husband died 10 years ago. She has settled well at the residential home and is quite popular with staff and other residents. She has no history of any other physical or psychiatric illness.

Mental state examination

She appears well dressed though there is some evidence of self-neglect. Her hair looks messy and her nails are dirty. She walks in with a stooped posture and takes slow shuffling steps. She has a prominent resting tremor when she sits down. Her head nods and her hands rhythmically move. She is cooperative, pleasant and establishes a good rapport. She reports her mood to be normal but on direct questioning she becomes tearful, saying she cannot help crying. Her affect is blunted. Her speech is soft and slow. There is no formal thought disorder. Cognitive examination reveals impairments in attention span, registration, recall, writing, construction and three-stage command. She has some insight into her condition, acknowledging her mobility problems and the need for treatment. However, she denies being disinhibited saying 'she was just being happy'.

Questions

- What is the differential diagnosis?
- What psychiatric complications of her treatment will you warn her about?

ANSWER 71

This woman has a diagnosis of Parkinson disease (PD), which is being treated with levodopa. She is now presenting with lability of mood associated with further deterioration of her cognitive abilities and her movement disorder. Differential diagnoses that need to be considered include the following:

- *Dementia:* risk of dementia may be increased up to three-fold in patients with PD. The majority of PD patients may have mild dementia characterized by memory problems and slow thinking, as may be likely in this case, and up to 20% may progress to severe dementia. The presence of cognitive changes must lead to referral to a psychiatrist or a neurologist to consider the possible diagnosis of dementia and its possible aetiology, including vascular dementia, Huntington disease, Hallervorden–Spatz disease, progressive supranuclear palsy and other rare conditions which may present with cognitive deterioration and movement disorder.
- *Depression:* is seen more commonly in PD (nearly 50%) than in other similar disabling conditions and is unrelated to duration of illness or to level of disability. PD may often present with symptoms of depression or anxiety. Females are more likely to be affected. Emotional insecurity, pessimism, lack of confidence in socializing or going out, poor motivation and increased concern about health are more common presenting symptoms.
- *Mania:* manic or other psychotic episodes are extremely rare in PD though psychotic depression may be seen in a small proportion of cases.
- *Iatrogenic:* psychosis, affective disorders, delirium and impulsive behaviours can occur as iatrogenic conditions secondary to overmedication with levodopa or anticholinergic medications. Impulsive behaviours can include hypersexuality, dopamine dysregulation syndrome with addiction to dopaminergic medications, as well as compulsive, addictive, repetitive or reward-seeking behaviours. Up to 14% of patients on dopamine agonists engage in pathological or harmful gambling. Up to 3% of PD patients seen in specialist clinics exhibit hypersexuality or dopamine dysregulation. Psychiatric side-effects are seen in 10% of cases increasing up to 60% in those on treatment over 6 years. Psychotic episodes, with delusions and hallucinations, may be precipitated in those with past history of psychosis or may occur as a new episode later in treatment. Visual hallucinations are more common (unlike schizophrenia where auditory hallucinations predominate) and insight is often preserved. They usually respond to reduction of antiparkinsonian treatment. Where this is not possible, treatment with atypical antipsychotics is appropriate, but with careful vigilance for worsening of motor symptoms. Mood disorders including mania, severe depression and anxiety can occur as treatment complications. Acute confusional states with disorientation and hallucinations may also be seen.

In this case, there are periods of low mood and tearfulness alternating with periods of hyperactivity, agitation and elated mood. This is most likely associated with on-off periods related to medication.

Key Points

- Psychiatric complications such as depression, mania, psychosis and cognitive disorders such as dementia or delirium are often associated with PD and/or secondary to medications used to treat PD.
- These complications increase with chronicity of illness and treatment and a high index of suspicion is needed to identify and effectively treat them.

CASE 72: SHE IS REFUSING TREATMENT. HER DECISION IS WRONG. SHE MUST BE MENTALLY ILL

History

A surgical colleague rings you up. He has a 75-year-old woman who needs an operation to remove a breast lump. The lump is malignant but is isolated, and there is no evidence of any local or distant spread. Your colleague explains he has told the woman that the operation is fairly straightforward and that after the operation she would be treated with radiotherapy. He states that she is saying she has no wish to have the operation. He is struggling to understand her decision because not having the operation reduces her chances of survival. He wants you to come and assess her because he feels she must have a mental illness which is rendering her incapable of making the right decision.

Questions

- Who should assess capacity?
- What conditions must be fulfilled for a person to have capacity to make a particular decision?
- What should happen here?

ANSWER 72

The Mental Capacity Act states that a person must be assumed to have capacity unless it is established that the person lacks capacity. A person suffering from a mental illness does not automatically lack capacity to make any decisions. Capacity has to be ascertained on an individual basis and for each situation where a decision is required. There is different legislation in England and Wales from Scotland (Adults with Incapacity, Scotland Act 2000) and Northern Ireland (Mental Capacity Act [Northern Ireland] 2016). Northern Ireland does not yet have such an act and draft legislation is out for consultation at the time of writing.

Assessment for capacity to make decisions regarding treatment must be made by the treating doctor. All health care professionals should be able to undertake capacity assessments.

! Mental Capacity Act considerations

- An individual lacks capacity to make a decision if, because of an impairment of or a disturbance in the functioning of the mind or brain they are
  - Unable to understand the information relevant to the decision.
  - Unable to retain the necessary information for long enough to make a decision.
  - Unable to use and weigh the information in order to arrive at a decision or unable to communicate his or her decision.
- Plain language should be used and enough information provided to enable a decision to be made. The quantity and quality of information should be proportionate to the complexity of the decision.
- The information needs to be retained by the person for long enough to give it proper consideration and weigh up the potential consequences.
- The patient should have the freedom to make the decision he or she wants and not be unduly pressured to come to a particular decision by others, for example, family members or professionals.

Capacity should be reviewed on a regular basis. Temporary impairment may improve. A person with a progressive illness such as dementia may lose capacity to make decisions.

Some patients will have previously recorded a decision about what they would decide if particular circumstances arise. Similarly, if the patient has given someone lasting power of attorney (previously enduring power of attorney) to make personal welfare decisions, the attorney may, subject to certain conditions, give or refuse consent to treatment on behalf of the patient. Doctors must, where practicable and appropriate, seek the views of family or carers, anyone who holds a lasting power of attorney to make personal welfare decisions or a deputy appointed by the Court of Protection to make decisions on behalf of the person.

The Mental Capacity Act is clear that anyone who has the care of a person who lacks capacity, and wilfully neglects or ill-treats that person, is guilty of an offence.

In this scenario the patient cannot be treated against her wishes unless it can be demonstrated that she lacks capacity to decide whether or not to have the treatment, and that the treatment is both necessary and in her best interests. She cannot be said to lack capacity just because her decision seems unwise to others or she does not agree with advice. However, if she fully understands the information given to her and can retain and use that information to make a balanced decision, she has capacity and her refusal of treatment must be respected.

Key Points

- Capacity can and should be assessed by any treating doctor.
- Capacity should be reviewed periodically.
- A patient who lacks capacity can be given treatment which is necessary and in the patient's best interests even if he or she refuses to consent.

CASE 73: LOW MOOD

History

You are asked to see a 69-year-old woman who complains of feeling constantly tired and not enjoying anything including her grandchildren. She sleeps for 8 hours or more but still never feels rested. She finds herself getting increasingly irritable and snappy with her 37-year-old daughter who is now living with her following the breakdown of her marriage. The daughter has two children ages 10 and 12 for whom the patient is having to provide care because her daughter is unable to manage this. The patient is finding the demands of her daughter, grandchildren and husband more and more difficult to cope with. She often forgets what needs to be done. Further questioning reveals that her daughter has agoraphobia and depression.

She has no previous history of mental health problems. She has hypertension which is well controlled.

Mental state examination

The woman looks tired and much older than her 69 years. She is obese and her dress is rather erratic. She has lots of layers of clothing and seems unaware that she has come in her slippers. She looks tired. Her speech is slow, flat and monosyllabic. She states she feels okay but she looks and sounds low. She does not have any active suicidal ideation but does question whether life is worth living. She feels hopeless about the circumstances she finds herself in. She has no hallucinations or formal thought disorder.

Questions

- What is the differential diagnosis?
- What investigations would be useful to do?
- How would you manage this situation?

ANSWER 73

The most likely diagnosis is depression secondary to her current life situation. However, there is a need to exclude an organic condition such as hypothyroidism, undiagnosed diabetes or alcohol misuse. Dementia will also need to be excluded given her memory loss.

Investigations

A full blood count would check for anaemia. If she is looking after everyone else her own care might be poor and she may well be anaemic (vitamin B_{12} deficiency may also need excluding). Thyroid function tests would exclude hypothyroidism, which can mimic depression. Liver function tests, blood sugar and urea and electrolytes would exclude systemic illnesses that may affect mood and coping. These are numerous and include, for example, neoplasia, diabetes, renal problems and liver problems.

If this woman's diagnosis is depression, she would benefit from antidepressant treatment and perhaps cognitive behaviour therapy (CBT). Given her current situation she might find it difficult to commit to CBT. A selective serotonin reuptake inhibitor (SSRI) such as citalopram or fluoxetine would be a reasonable choice. Use of medication needs to be carefully monitored as the elderly are more sensitive to drug side-effects. Ensuring that her daughter is receiving treatment in her own right may also help. Practical support from social services, family or the community is also likely to be helpful. Careful consideration must be given to the welfare of her grandchildren for whom she has responsibility, as her illness may impact on her ability to care for them.

Depression in older adults may present differently than in younger people. For example, low energy levels and reduced motivation may be presenting features rather than reported sadness. Worry about money, health or family members is not uncommon. Physical complaints may also be the presenting feature including headaches or other aches and pains. They may see it as related to getting older and are less likely to go to their doctor.

Common features of depression in the elderly

- Unexplained or aggravated aches and pains
- Hopelessness
- Helplessness
- Anxiety and worries
- Memory problems
- Loss of pleasure
- Lack of personal care
- Irritability
- Loss of motivation and energy

Key Points

- Depression is more likely with medical problems in the elderly.
- Feelings of sadness may not be identified or commented on by the elderly.
- The elderly may fail to seek help in their own right for their mental health problems.

CASE 74: MY WIFE IS AN IMPOSTOR

History

A 68-year-old retired aircraft engineer presents to his general practitioner (GP) asking for help in removing an impostor from his home. He goes on to tell the GP that his wife was replaced by someone else 2 weeks ago but that this impostor is very clever and has managed to take on his wife's appearance, voice and mannerisms. He refuses to be in the same room as the impostor and frequently shouts at her to leave and return his real wife. He has also called the police to ask them to eject her from his home. His wife is distraught by this behaviour and despite her pleas and the intervention of other family members the patient refuses to believe that she is really his wife.

A year ago he had a coronary artery bypass graft and has done well since this operation. He continues to have hyperlipidaemia, hypertension and type 2 diabetes mellitus. He is an ex-smoker, who stopped smoking a year ago, having previously smoked 40 cigarettes per day for nearly 50 years. He has no other past medical history of note and no previous psychiatric history. There is no history of alcohol or substance abuse.

He and his wife have been married for 40 years and have three grown-up children. There is no family history of psychiatric illness.

Mental state examination

He presents as a well-kempt elderly man who looks older than his chronological age. He makes normal eye contact. His speech is slow and repetitive and on occasions there are long pauses during which it appears he is struggling to find the appropriate word. His mood is normal and there is no evidence of depression. He is adamant that his wife has been replaced by an impostor but is unable to explain why or how this occurred. There is no formal thought disorder or hallucinations. On cognitive testing he scores 24 out of 30 on the Mini Mental State Examination (MMSE) with particular deficits in the areas of registration and language.

There is no abnormality on physical examination.

Questions

- What psychopathological syndrome is being described?
- Why is detailed cognitive examination important in this case?

ANSWER 74

This is a description of Capgras syndrome – a rare condition in which the patient believes that an impostor who has taken on a similar appearance has replaced a family member or close acquaintance. Capgras syndrome is more properly referred to as Capgras delusion as it is a particular type of delusional disorder (delusional misrepresentation of personal identity). It is most commonly seen in schizophrenia but a third of cases are thought to be due to organic pathology such as brain injury or dementia.

! Other rare delusional disorders

- *Fregoli delusion:* a belief that another person disguises himself or herself as several people.
- *Delusional misidentification:* this is a catch-all phrase for Capgras syndrome, Fregoli delusion and other misidentification syndromes such as the belief in a doppelganger (or double).
- *Cotard syndrome:* a delusion that the person is dead or that a part of the person is dead or does not exist.
- *Erotomania:* the belief that another person (often of higher status) is in love with the sufferer.

This man has a number of risk factors for cerebrovascular accident and vascular dementia (i.e. hyperlipidaemia, hypertension, type 2 diabetes mellitus and ischaemic heart disease). Given this and the high prevalence of organic aetiology in Capgras syndrome it is important to thoroughly assess his cognitive functioning. In addition to cognitive testing using a tool such as the MMSE or Addenbrooke's Cognitive Examination (ACE) it would be appropriate to refer this man for brain imaging. Consideration may also need to be given to referring him to a neuropsychologist for more detailed cognitive assessment.

It is interesting to note that patients with this presentation have an intact ability to recognize faces (i.e. they do not have prosopagnosia). It is thought that they do not experience an appropriate emotional response when they do recognize the face of the person they believe has been replaced by an impostor. From this it is hypothesized that it is the lack of an appropriate emotional response that leads the patient into believing that there is something odd about the person from which develops the delusion that the person is really an impostor.

Key Points

- Delusional misinterpretation of personal identity may be indicative of organic pathology.
- It is important to perform detailed cognitive examination in all such cases.

CASE 75: MARKED TREMOR, GETTING WORSE

History

A 75-year-old man presents worried that he has recently developed quite a marked tremor and nothing he can do helps control it. He has no other concerns and is currently well. The man has a long established diagnosis of bipolar disorder, which has been well controlled with lithium. His medication was recently changed.

Mental state examination

The man is cooperative and communicative with good eye contact. His speech is normal. His mood is objectively and subjectively stable. He does not express any ideas of self-harm. There is no evidence of psychosis. He is orientated in time, place and person and there is no cognitive impairment.

Physical examination

The man looks well and there is nothing of note except a marked coarse tremor. The tremor is not rhythmic and is present at rest and when he attempts a task. There is no indication of any cogwheel rigidity or lack of facial expressions.

Questions

- What is the differential diagnosis?
- What are the signs of lithium toxicity?
- How should lithium toxicity be managed?
- How can the potential for lithium toxicity be minimized?

ANSWER 75

The most likely diagnosis would be lithium toxicity but other disorders such as Parkinson disease should be excluded.

People who are taking lithium for bipolar disorder may develop lithium toxicity because there is only a small difference between a therapeutic serum lithium level and a toxic level. Patients therefore need to have regular blood tests that measure serum lithium levels. In order for this to be meaningful, blood should be taken 10–14 hours after the previous dose. The usual therapeutic range is between 0.4 and 1 mmol/L.

Many adverse effects of lithium are dose related. However, taking non-steroidal anti-inflammatory drugs (NSAIDs) in combination with lithium can interfere with lithium excretion. This can lead to a dangerous buildup of lithium levels. If NSAIDs are essential the dosage of lithium may need to be reduced and regular blood tests to check lithium levels remain necessary.

Mild gastrointestinal symptoms, fine hand tremor, mild thirst and polyuria and a metallic taste in the mouth are all recognized side-effects which can occur when serum levels are within the therapeutic range. Lithium toxicity is a potentially life-threatening condition and is usually associated with serum levels greater than 1.5 mmol/L but can occur at lower serum levels.

! Symptoms and signs of lithium toxicity

- Blurred vision
- Worsening gastrointestinal symptoms (anorexia, diarrhoea, vomiting)
- Muscle weakness, drowsiness, ataxia, coarse tremor and muscle twitching

Severe toxicity (serum levels above 2 mmol/L) can lead to

- Hyperreflexia, disorientation, seizures, syncope, renal failure, nystagmus, circulatory failure, coma and death

Many people may endure mild side-effects in order to take an effective dosage. However, if symptoms become worse (or new symptoms develop), lithium toxicity should be suspected.

! Be alerted:

- Lithium levels >1.5 mmol/L (>2.0 mmol/L may be associated with serious toxicity).
- Lithium toxicity should also be suspected at 'therapeutic' levels in compromised patients with relevant symptoms.

Treatment for toxic levels of lithium

The treatment for lithium toxicity depends on a few factors, including the level of lithium in the blood. If the level in the blood is very high, dialysis can be helpful. Stopping lithium for a while may be necessary, although a dose reduction may be adequate in mild cases. Rehydration can also be helpful.

Preventing lithium toxicity

Patients need to be properly educated on the symptoms of toxicity so they can identify them early and also be aware of the need for close monitoring. Regular fluid intake is important as dehydration increases risk of toxicity as do crash diets. Doses cannot be skipped and made up later, so careful compliance is key.

Key Points

- Lithium toxicity can be fatal so needs prompt attention.
- Careful monitoring and patient education should prevent severe toxicity.
- Be aware of interactions with other medications.

CASE 76: HE CAN'T SIT STILL

History

A 7-year-old boy appears in the accident and emergency department having banged his head after falling from a garage roof. He vomited once after this but has not become unconscious or had any loss of power or sensation. He has had no other neurological problems on systematic enquiry. His parents are with him. They say that he has always been very active and ask if he can be seen by someone who might check him out. He has a normal night's sleep but is very active when awake. He rarely stays on task and does not finish things that he starts. He has always flitted from toy to toy when playing. His teachers report to the parents that he is a fidget, up and down out of his chair, and that he has very poor concentration. He calls answers out despite being reminded not to and has great difficulty waiting in a queue. He is easily distracted by things outside the window or in other parts of the classroom. This is much the same at home. If he takes anything to school he often loses it and has had to have three new coats in the last year because previous ones have gone missing. Even when watching favoured television programmes he will be up and down out of the chair, and in and out of the room.

Questions

- What is the most likely cause of his problems?
- What interventions are available?

ANSWER 76

It is likely that this boy has attention deficit hyperactivity disorder (ADHD). This is a *Diagnostic and Statistical Manual of Mental Disorders, 5th Edition* (*DSM-5*) diagnosis characterized by pervasively poor ability to concentrate (i.e. not in one situation only), impulsivity, distractibility and overactivity. These should be present in greater severity and frequency than that found developmentally. While all small children can be distractible in some settings, in ADHD this continues from infancy and remains present at primary school.

There are two main types: ADHD predominately inattentive and ADHD mixed type. The latter includes all four main symptom groups of attention/concentration, impulsivity, distractibility and overactivity. The former includes the other three main symptoms but not overactivity. There is a theoretical third group, ADHD predominately overactive, but this is rarely found since most of the overactive children also have the other difficulties. The World Health Organization uses the term *hyperkinetic disorder*, and this maps onto the combined type of ADHD from *DSM-5*. ADHD has a significant impact on social and educational functioning.

In the differential it is important to consider attachment disorders. Young children who are neglected or abused emotionally, and young children who have consistently poor experiences of parenting, can develop attachment disorders which have an impact on behaviour and social relationships. One of the subtypes is a disinhibited attachment disorder, which can look similar to ADHD. Many parents mistake conduct disorders and oppositional defiant disorder for ADHD. This is because ADHD is a risk factor for behavioural problems, and so children with ADHD often go on to develop conduct disorder. However, the reverse is not true. Being true to the diagnosis of ADHD, it is important to make sure that children do not end up on unnecessary or inappropriate treatments. Organic problems also need to be considered including epilepsy, fragile X syndrome and neurodegenerative disorders. Children who have dyslexia are also at high risk of classroom failure, and concomitant behaviours. This should always be checked.

The main treatments for ADHD are educational and behavioural interventions through parenting programmes and advice to teachers. Some children require extra help in school. Where a child is at risk of social failure, educational failure or family breakdown then medication with stimulants such as methylphenidate or dexamfetamine are appropriate. This dramatically improves concentration in children. It is not a diagnostic test because it improves concentration in most children, but can be particularly helpful for children with ADHD. Some psychiatrists prescribe this for school days only, while if symptoms are severe the child may be prescribed the medication 7 days a week. Drug holidays at least every year are helpful during summer breaks to review progress and check the need for ongoing medication. A variety of second-line medications have been used if stimulants are not effective, including clonidine, atomoxetine, and tricyclics. Many young people's symptoms improve with age. Good services have a range of psychosocial interventions including specialist parenting groups, skills programmes for children and adolescents and advice about environmental management (e.g. sensory aspects). This empowers children and young people to live with their neurodevelopmental difficulties and develop coping strategies that allow them to come off medication in adolescence.

Key Points

- Genetic factors are known to be important in ADHD.
- Environmental factors such as parenting can influence outcome.
- For severe ADHD, stimulant medication is used alongside psychosocial interventions (parenting support and behavioural and educational interventions).

CASE 77: SOCIALLY ISOLATED

History

A 12-year-old girl is brought by her parents to the general practitioner (GP) surgery. Her mother is concerned that in year 7 at secondary school she has no friends. She spends most of her time in the library or walking around the playground. She has never had many friends although there was one boy in year 6 who came to her house sometimes to play on the computer. They took it in turns, but her mother recalls that they rarely spoke to each other and when they did it was to discuss the details of the game. Sometimes her daughter would leave her friend playing on her own and go and do something in another room. She is not very good at responding when others in the family are hurt. She will stop and watch or carry on what she is doing. Her father gave the example of him banging his head on a sharp corner on her ninth birthday. He swore and had tears in his eyes. His daughter asked, without much emotion, why his 'eyes were wet'. Her mother describes that she has been doing reasonably well with schoolwork, and is in top set for sciences and mathematics, although in mathematics the teacher has fed back that she is resistant to doing things the way the teacher wants, preferring to do things her own way. She is very interested in electric fans and has a collection of at least 20. She is also very knowledgeable about aeroplanes and can talk at length and in detail about various makes across history. Her teacher says that she sometimes takes things literally. Once when the teacher said, 'take your seats', she picked her seat up and asked where she should take it. She will tell other children if what they are doing is against the rules, and is unpopular as a result. She has always struggled greatly with role-play activities but can be very creative. She paints repeated pictures of ponies and has hundreds of them. When she comes in from school she goes round the house checking that certain objects are in the 'right' place and this takes about 15 minutes. She has no history of delay in motor or language acquisition milestones.

Mental state examination

In the surgery her eye contact is poor, and she has a tendency to turn to her mother when the GP asks her a question. She is smartly dressed in a tracksuit, and noticeably has no zips or buttons (her mother says she also has to cut labels off as her daughter does not like them). There is no evidence of any psychomotor retardation, or any psychotic phenomena. She says that she is happy and has no problems. When asked who her friends are she lists her teaching assistant and her mother. There is no evidence of psychosis or depressive illness.

Questions

- What is the likely diagnosis?
- What possible interventions may help?

The DSM5 American Psychiatric Association has recently dropped the term Asperger syndrome in favour of autism spectrum disorder mild, moderate and severe; but there is a lot of discontent about this system from both users (who like the term Asperger syndrome) and from clinicians. The World Health Organization system (currently ICD-10) continues to use the diagnostic term Asperger syndrome and it remains widely used in many countries.

ANSWER 77

The most likely diagnosis is Asperger syndrome. This is on the autism spectrum of conditions, and involves social reciprocity problems, delay in imagination skills and repetitive or stereotyped interests and behaviours. It is different from autism in that there is no delay in language acquisition and no cognitive delay (IQ below 70). Although her language acquisition was normal, she does have problems with the pragmatics of language and is likely to take things literally and have problems with abstract thinking. She is also likely to have conversational reciprocity problems. She has some 'mind blindness' where she is poor at understanding other people's emotions, for example, when her father was hurt. She clearly has a very limited understanding of friendship, and has peer relationship problems. She also has eye contact problems. She has some unusual preoccupations including fans and an intense preoccupation with aeroplanes. Although preoccupations themselves are not necessarily diagnostic, they are often present.

Differential diagnosis includes depression, generalized anxiety, separation anxiety or social anxiety disorder of childhood. Asperger syndrome is lifelong, whereas anxiety and depression have an onset that may be related to life events such as family breakdown, bereavement, trauma, stress or significant change. Social anxiety is not usually accompanied by delay in imaginative development or the presence of repetitive and stereotyped patterns of behaviour. Some clinicians think that girls on the autism spectrum may present differently from boys (e.g. with more protected imagination skills and/or less repetitive and restricted behaviours), but good research needs to be done to clarify this. Obsessive-compulsive disorder (OCD) should be considered but would not normally have the range of other problems such as social reciprocity difficulties and imagination delay. Also, preoccupations or intense interests in Asperger syndrome are usually enjoyed, and therefore different from the resisted obsessions and compulsions of OCD, and so are termed preoccupations rather than obsessions. Extreme shyness in an otherwise healthy child should be considered but would not usually involve the significant theory of mind delays (mind blindness). Some children have socio-emotional delay that can mimic Asperger syndrome because of early life social or communicative deprivation. Examples of this would be deaf children born into hearing families where early life communication is poor, or children in orphanages in developing countries who have little interaction with others. Emotionally abused or neglected children can also have poor empathy and odd social behaviour depending on what they have experienced.

Making the diagnosis and getting it right is important as it directs parents, carers and teachers towards helpful interventions. Diagnosis can be aided by diagnostic interviews (such as the Autism Diagnostic Interview [Revised] or the Diagnostic Interview for Social and Communication Disorders) and interactive assessments (such as the Autism Diagnostic Observation Schedule [ADOS-2]). The new *Diagnostic and Statistical Manual of Mental Disorders, Fifth Edition* (*DSM-5*; American Psychiatric Association) system of classification has dispensed with the diagnostic category Asperger Disorder (the equivalent to the World Health Organisation's [WHO] Asperger Syndrome), in favour of Autism Spectrum Disorder Mild, Moderate and Severe. The WHO is still considering its new *International Classification of Diseases, 11th Revision* (*ICD-11*) system.

Children with Asperger syndrome need extra support in school. While some children with autism may need a special school, those with Asperger syndrome would usually be supported in mainstream school. Parent training programmes have been shown to be helpful in improving developmental pathways. Group work for the child including daily living skill work, independence work and support for social interaction may also help. Individual work from parents and teachers can use a variety of books and computer programmes designed to teach skills and abilities that children with Asperger syndrome may find it hard to pick up intuitively. This includes learning social rules, learning to read body language and facial expressions and learning social problem-solving skills. Occasionally medication such as selective serotonin reuptake inhibitors may be helpful for intense compulsions or ritualized behaviour, although there needs to be further research to give a more robust evidence base for their use. Children and young people with Asperger syndrome can be happy and successful given the right support and environment, so education and career pathways are very important.

Allowing them to develop their interests and supporting them in their productive interests can be helpful and rewarding.

Key Points

- Asperger syndrome is similar to autism but with an IQ above 70 and without language acquisition delay.
- Mind blindness (delay in the development of theory of mind skills) is a core feature.
- Interventions designed to support development and learning of socio-emotional skills are helpful.

CASE 78: KILLED HIS FRIEND'S HAMSTER AND IN TROUBLE ALL THE TIME

History

A 14-year-old boy presents to casualty with cuts on his hand that require stitches. It transpires that the injury was sustained in a fight with a friend because he killed the hamster of his friend's younger sibling. He has shown no remorse and appears amused by the distress he has caused. He rarely attends school, usually preferring to play truant with peers. When he does go to school, he often gets into trouble for threatening behaviour and for answering back. His mother feels she has no control over her son and that his aggressive behaviour is escalating. His mother also states that he runs around with a bad group who are probably engaged in vandalism and theft. She states that her son can be very moody and has more recently been erratic in his behaviour. She says she thinks he is often restless and cannot sleep at night. She hears him wandering round the house but when she has tried to talk to him he tells her to mind her own business. He has had no regular contact with his father who has spent spells in prison.

Mental state examination

You are faced with a hostile, sullen teenager who is verbally abusive and makes poor eye contact. He is uncooperative and impatient, demanding his injury be dealt with immediately so he can leave. He is also abusive towards his mother when she tries to interject. He denies feeling low in mood and has not tried to harm himself. During your interview there is no evidence that he is being bothered by hallucinations and does not come across as thought disordered. He is orientated in time, place and person.

Questions

- What causes might you consider to explain this boy's presentation?
- How would you manage this case?

ANSWER 78

It is worth formulating this child's difficulties in a multi-axial way. The differential diagnosis is conduct disorder, oppositional defiant disorder, attention deficit hyperactivity disorder, anxiety, depression, social phobia, substance misuse, learning disability and any combination of these disorders. He may have callous unemotional traits. As with most child mental health problems, conduct disorder has a multifactorial aetiology. Exposure to the antisocial behaviour of a caregiver is a particularly important risk factor. Children with conduct disorder appear to be overrepresented in lower socioeconomic groups.

! Multi-axial classification (*International Classification of Diseases, Tenth Revision* [*ICD-10*])

- Axis 1: Mental health diagnosis
- Axis 2: Developmental
- Axis 3: Intellectual
- Axis 4: Organic/physical
- Axis 5: Psychosocial

While most clinicians are keen to avoid pathologizing young people with diagnostic labels, the classification systems recognize that certain patterns of severe behaviour have significant consequences for child, family, community and prognosis. Conduct disorder is a repetitive and persistent pattern of behaviours in which the rights of others are violated or there is age-inappropriate violation of societal norms lasting at least 6 months. The behaviours include unusually severe and frequent outbursts that are developmentally inappropriate, argumentative, not compliant with authority, hostile and angry, untruthful and may include aggression, physical cruelty to animals, vandalism, truancy, criminal activity and bullying. This list is not exhaustive.

While *ICD-10* defines conduct disorder in terms of *socialized*, *unsocialized* or *confined to the home context*, more recent research suggests a subdivision of two subtypes: *childhood-onset type* which has onset before the age of 10 years, and *adolescent-onset type* with no conduct problems before this age. This is reflected in the *Diagnostic and Statistical Manual of Mental Disorders* (*DSM*) criteria which differ from those of *ICD*. The childhood-onset type is often very difficult to treat. It is long-standing and is usually associated with psychosocial adversity and poor parenting. It has a worse prognosis than short-lived adolescent problems, where behaviours may be reflective of adolescent development such as risk taking and experimenting (e.g. with drugs). In many this behaviour does not persist. Harming animals is a particularly worrying feature. In general, most children and young people with conduct disorder do not go on to become antisocial adults, but most antisocial adults have had conduct problems when younger.

Conduct disorder is a difficult disorder to treat and there are high levels of co-morbidity such as low mood. This should be excluded. There is little evidence to justify the use of medication to control aggression. For childhood-onset type, parenting programmes should be used as early as practicable, as negative ineffective parenting may perpetuate the problems. Family therapy, support and behaviour modification may help. The young man may benefit from a positive relationship with a male. Youth groups can sometimes provide healthy peer influences and role models.

The acute management would involve dealing with his hand injury. Being sympathetic but not allowing him to push boundaries may help him feel contained and improve his engagement with you. A referral to a parenting support service or child mental health services as an outpatient may allow the family to discuss any issues that need addressing.

Key Points

- Conduct disorder often has co-morbidity with other disorders so it is important to exclude and treat co-existing disorders.
- To date conduct disorder is difficult to treat and has a relatively poor prognosis, particularly when onset is in childhood, behaviours are long-standing and when peers and family demonstrate similar behaviours.

CASE 79: I ONLY FAINTED: DON'T FUSS AND LEAVE ME ALONE

History

A 17-year-old girl is admitted to casualty having fainted during a games lesson at school. She is embarrassed by the fuss she has caused and insists she is okay. She skipped breakfast and says she is now fine and would like to be discharged. She denies any problems with her health. She reluctantly admits that her periods are less regular than they had been. She had menarche at the age of 13 but over the last 6 months has only had two periods. She is not sexually active. She is doing extremely well at school in her AS subjects having achieved 10 A stars at General Certificate of Secondary Education (GCSE) 6 months ago. Her parents recently separated but she feels they have minimized the impact on her and her younger two siblings.

Physical examination

She looks very tired and has slightly sunken cheeks. Her clothing is very baggy and ill fitting. Her fingers are tinged blue and she feels cold to touch. She has fine downy hair on her arms. Her height is 160 cm and weight is 42 kg, giving her a body mass index (BMI) of 16.4. There is no evidence of other serious mental illness.

! BMI

BMI is a standardized ratio of weight to height, and is often used as a general indicator of health. BMI can be calculated by dividing the weight (in kilograms) by the square of the height (in metres). A BMI between 18.5 and 24.9 is considered normal for most adults. Higher BMIs may indicate that an individual is overweight or obese.

Investigations

	Levels	*Reference range*
Haemoglobin	12.8 g/dL	11.7–15.7 g/dL
White cell count	8.8 × 10^9/L	3.5–11.0 × 10^9/L
Platelets	280 × 10^9/L	150–440 × 10^9/L
Sodium	139 mmol/L	135–145 mmol/L
Potassium	3.4 mmol/L	3.5–5.0 mmol/l
Urea	7.4 mmol/L	2.5–6.7 mmol/L
Creatinine	75 µmol/L	70–120 µmol/L

Questions

- What is the differential diagnosis?
- How would you manage this case?

ANSWER 79

The most likely diagnosis is anorexia nervosa. Differential diagnosis includes organic conditions (unlikely but needs exclusion) and depression. Phobia of foodstuffs (e.g. solid food) and obsessive-compulsive disorder could also be considered. For anorexia to be diagnosed there must be weight loss (or in children a lack of weight gain). The limitation of the BMI is that it may overestimate body fat in those with muscular build and may underestimate body fat in those who have lost muscle fat. It is also less reliable in younger teenagers. The weight loss is self-induced often by avoiding eating but especially by avoiding fattening foods. Associated with poor food intake, there may be obsessive behaviour around preparation of food for others. There may also be associated vomiting and laxative abuse to ensure that no weight is gained. Vomiting may lead to hypokalaemia which can be dangerous particularly if it changes rapidly. Excessive exercise may also be present. Amenorrhoea may be present in those who have started their periods, as the body seeks to conserve resources. A key feature is that those with the disorder have distorted cognition that they are too fat with real fear of gaining weight and becoming fat. This is despite the evidence that they are underweight and often dangerously so. The belief that they are too fat often has a delusional quality but there are no other features of psychosis. However, prolonged starvation itself has an impact on cognitive functioning. Once weight loss is in progress, immunological and hormonal factors may play a role in a malignant spiral down and maintenance of anorexia nervosa. The mortality for anorexia is high at around 5% (and 0.5% per year). Anorexia occurs significantly more in females (around 100 females to 1 male) and is more common in Western cultures, but can occur in all cultures. It is tending to occur in younger and younger children. The aetiology is multi-factorial and it is thought that media representations of women play a major role in the disorder. Prognosis is worse for onset before 11 years of age and in adulthood. Around 50% of individuals with anorexia will recover, but others will continue to have problems.

It is important to undertake a thorough assessment and a corroborative history will be important. Acute management needs to make sure she is medically safe, so rehydration would be the first step as she is dehydrated. Longer-term management will include referral to specialist Child and Adolescent Mental Health Services (CAMHS) or an eating disorder team (depending on local arrangements). The priority will be to work towards gradual and sustained weight gain and cognitive behaviour therapy (CBT), which works towards changing their relationship with food. There is good evidence that in children under 14 years of age family therapy is effective and is the treatment of choice. Antidepressants may be required for those who also have a strong affective component. Prolonged starvation takes its toll on the body and will cause physical side effects that warrant attention.

! Medical complications of anorexia nervosa

- Amenorrhoea
- Fatigue and dizziness
- Intolerance to cold
- Lanugo
- Constipation and abdominal pain
- Loss of menstrual periods
- Lack of energy and weakness
- Feeling cold all the time
- Dry, yellowish skin

Longer-term medical complications of anorexia may be hair loss, osteoporosis, tooth decay, damage to the oesophagus or larynx from acid reflux, stunted growth, infertility, heart problems, kidney failure and death.

Key Points

- Anorexia often presents through physical complications.
- Anorexia carries a high mortality.

CASE 80: CUTTING ON THE FOREARMS

History

A 16-year-old girl presents after being in a car accident where a car drove into the back of the car that her mother was driving. This happened on a motorway slip road the previous day. Having initially thought there were no injuries, she has woken up with pain and stiffness in her neck and a sore right wrist. She thinks she may have knocked it on the dashboard. She attends the general practitioner (GP) surgery and you examine her.

Mental state examination

On examination she has no evidence of any fractures, no neurological symptoms or signs on history or examination. You diagnose whiplash and recommend simple analgesia, a neck collar and arrange physiotherapy. On examination you notice multiple new and old transverse scars on her forearms hidden underneath a long-sleeved jumper. On further discussion the girl explains that she has been cutting herself on a regular basis to relieve stress for about 18 months. Some of the scarring is deep. On examination of her spine there are several linear scars on her lower outer back extending round to her abdomen.

Questions

- What reasons are there for this form of self-harm that you should consider when taking a further history?
- What aspects of risk assessment should you consider?

ANSWER 80

There are various things the GP will need to ask about. It will be necessary to rule out *depression*.

Factors to ask about to rule out depression

- Mood
- Levels of energy
- Sleep patterns
- Appetite
- Ability to enjoy oneself (anhedonia is loss of pleasure in things previously enjoyed)
- Concentration
- Loss of interest in or withdrawal from everyday activities
- Lethargy
- Feelings of guilt
- Hopelessness or low self-worth
- Irritability
- Ideas of self-harm or suicidal thoughts or intent

It is always important in any situation where there has been self-harm or low mood to enquire about past history of self-harm, and thoughts of suicide. This should be approached sensitively and gently with questions like: 'Do you ever think that life is not worth living?' 'Would you ever do anything about these thoughts?' 'Have you any particular plans?' (see Case 33).

However, many young people who cut are not depressed, and the GP will need to ask about other things. Is the young person cutting because she has obsessional thoughts or ruminations that only go away temporarily when she cuts (obsessive-compulsive disorder [OCD])? Is the cutting maladaptive care-seeking behaviour? Some young people stumble across this when they cut once in response to a stressful event and it elicits a lot of support or kudos from a peer group or caring professional or family member. Occasionally several members of the same social group may cut and do this in a mutually supportive or competitive way. It can also occur in a socialized context, where several school friends are cutting as part of a subcultural group that is associated with certain types of music or subcultural viewpoints. Young people may also cut to avoid a predicament, such as a dreaded examination in a perfectionistic child who feels unprepared, or impending return home to an abusive parent. The cutting may be a mechanism for emotional regulation where feelings of guilt are acted out, or trapped emotions (such as anger) are internalized and expressed against the self.

Risk assessment

Good risk-assessment tools consider risks of

- Self-harm
- Suicide
- Exploitation
- Abuse
- Neglect
- Harm to others

This young woman should be referred to a child mental health team who can more formally assess what is going on and what interventions to offer. The treatment will depend on the reasons for the self-harm, and will range from no 'treatment' to group, family or individual therapy (e.g. cognitive behaviour therapy [CBT]). Where risk is assessed as low and where the young person does not want treatment (e.g. with a subcultural desire to cut without other signs of mental illness) then follow-up may not be appropriate. At the other end of the spectrum, serious cutting with intent to commit suicide should be taken seriously, and where the young person does not want treatment the Mental Health Act should be considered.

Key Points

- There are many different causes for self-harm behaviour and careful assessment is necessary to establish the most appropriate treatment.
- Parental consent can be used for minors refusing treatment.
- It is commonly thought that the Mental Health Act can only be used with adults. This is not the case. The Mental Health Act can be used with any age if appropriate.

CASE 81: FEELINGS OF GUILT

History

A 15-year-old girl presents with a 4-month history of feelings of being a failure and hopelessness. She is overwhelmed by feelings of guilt that she is a burden to her family. She thinks her parents are unaware of how bad she feels as she has not shared her feelings with them because she does not want them to worry.

She has been struggling with her schoolwork which has declined over the last 4 months. Her concentration is very poor and she has struggled to complete work in class or at home. She has lost some friends who have found it a misery to be around her. Up until about 6 months ago she was doing well in school with a good group of friends. She used to be actively involved in school activities but this has now fallen away as have social activities with friends at the weekend. Sometimes she will force herself to spend time with friends because she feels guilty about letting people down, but does not enjoy the activity and feels even worse after it.

She does not sleep well. She lies in bed worrying about everything that has happened and worrying about what she has done wrong. When she does fall asleep she will wake after a short time. She dreads waking up in the morning and facing the day ahead. At other times she may sleep for long periods but feels no more rested. Her appetite is poor and she has lost some weight.

She has regular thoughts of self-harm but is torn by her mixed feelings. Part of her feels that if she did harm herself her family would be upset so that prevents her from carrying out her thoughts. At other times she feels it would be in her family's interests if she did end her life so she could stop being a burden. She does not see the situation improving. She has thoughts of taking an overdose when no one else is at home.

Mental state examination

She is casually dressed and struggles to make eye contact. She is cooperative but often struggles to answer your questions. She cannot be distracted by small talk. Her speech is slow and laboured. She states that she feels low and she looks and sounds depressed. She has regular and persistent thoughts regarding self-harm but has not yet acted out these feelings. She does not see much hope for the future. There is no evidence of psychosis. She is orientated in time, place and person.

Questions

- What is the most likely diagnosis?
- How would you manage this girl?

ANSWER 81

The most likely diagnosis is moderate to severe depression. Features of depression include biological symptoms. Look for marked loss of interest or pleasure in usually pleasurable activities, lack of emotional responses to situations that usually would evoke a response, diurnal mood variation, sleep disturbance (young people may not get the early morning waking associated with depression in adults, and often find that they sleep more but still do not feel rested), poor appetite and/or weight loss (again young people may eat more), psychomotor retardation and agitation. Biological symptoms are less consistent in young people. Associated with these will be low mood and inability to concentrate. The young person may experience lack of confidence, poor self-esteem, negative feelings (such as worthlessness, guilt) and self-harm ideation. Moderate depression has greater severity and often a greater number of symptoms. Mild and moderate depression do not have psychotic features (see Case 83).

Everybody learns lists in different ways. The symptoms of depression can be thought of as computer MAC GAMES, with letters standing for the 12 main symptoms mentioned in *International Classification of Diseases, Tenth Revision* (*ICD-10*): depressed *m*ood for at least 2 weeks, *a*nhedonia, poor *c*oncentration, *g*uilty feelings, *a*ppetite disturbance, abnormal *m*ovements, low *e*nergy and then the 5 *S*'s of low *s*elf-esteem, thoughts of suicide/self-harm, sleep disturbance, reduced sex drive and somatization.

! *ICD-10* categories of non-psychotic depression

- F33 Recurrent Depressive Disorder
- F32 Depressive Episode
- F32.0 Mild Depressive Episode (4 from 12 symptoms)
- F32.1 Moderate Depressive Episode (6 from 12 symptoms)
- F32.2 Severe Depressive Episode (8 from 12) Without Psychotic Symptoms

Depression is more common in girls but it may be that it presents with more aggressive and hostile behaviour in males. It is less common before adolescence. There is some genetic loading, but in many cases the social disadvantage that is experienced by parents leading to depression is also experienced by their children.

An initial assessment which includes a detailed risk assessment is necessary. This girl is at moderate risk of harming herself given the feelings of being a burden and not having shared how bad she has felt. It would also be useful to get a parental history as they may provide some useful insights into her pre-morbid personality.

She would best be managed by individual counselling and medication. Medication is not as efficacious in adolescents. Certain serotonin reuptake inhibitors such as fluoxetine have the best evidence base. Once her mood has lifted and she is more amenable, cognitive behaviour therapy (CBT) or interpersonal therapy would be useful to help her manage both her negative feelings and feelings of guilt. Given her age it is also important to engage her parents so that they can provide appropriate support and also another perspective.

Key Points

- Depression is relatively common in adolescents.
- A high proportion of depression in adolescence abates with time and change in circumstances.
- Mild and moderate depression may be effectively treated with CBT and/or interpersonal therapy.
- Severe depression may need to be managed using the serotonin reuptake inhibitor, fluoxetine.

CASE 82: INTENSE FEELINGS OF WORTHLESSNESS

History

A 15-year-old girl is presented by her mother. The girl has a 6-month history of becoming increasingly withdrawn and irritable. She is barely eating and wants to sleep all the time, complaining of being tired. She is no longer attending school as she cannot concentrate and cannot cope with having to deal with other people. She used to be a high achiever at school but recently her work has declined. Over the last few weeks her parents have become even more concerned as at times the girl appears to be talking to herself and has become acutely distressed and tearful for no obvious reason. Her mother reports that all was reasonably well up until 6 months ago. There were a number of family losses just before that time but she feels her daughter managed reasonably well. There is no particular family history of note. The mother is not aware of any substance misuse.

Mental state examination

The girl avoids eye contact and is non-communicative. She has psychomotor retardation but no waxy flexibility. She is dishevelled with uncombed hair and is wearing her bed clothes. She is socially detached. Her speech is slow and almost retarded. She appears not to hear what you are saying and often struggles to formulate a response. She says she feels 'okay' but is convinced that she does not deserve to live. When pushed she states she is worthless and this is confirmed by berating voices which continually confirm that self-belief of worthlessness. She avoids answering your questions about whether she has considered self-harm or whether she has made any attempts or plans. She is also convinced that everyone agrees with the voices. She is able to provide evidence of her worthlessness in aspects of her parents' responses to her. She is orientated in person but not aware of the time of day or the day of the week. She is aware she is at home but not sure of why she is seeing you.

Questions

- What is the differential diagnosis?
- How would you manage this situation?

ANSWER 82

The most likely diagnosis is depression with psychotic features. Differential diagnosis would include bipolar disorder, organic psychosis, schizophrenia and substance misuse. However the delusions of worthlessness and derogatory hallucinations make depression with psychosis more likely. The features of depression in young people have been outlined in Case 81.

The immediate concern would be the high risk of this girl attempting to take her own life. Although self-harm in adolescents is very common, completed suicide is not. However, the risk rises when there is a mental illness. The fact that she feels she is worthless together with her psychotic features make this a high-risk situation. Her detachment is also worrying. The acute management requires a risk assessment. Inpatient care may need to be considered especially if she is evasive about her self-harm ideation. It is important to check mental state across time as this can vary greatly in teenagers. It is likely that she will need treatment with serotonin reuptake inhibiting antidepressants (such as fluoxetine). Given the extent of her psychosis, antipsychotic medication will also be required. Aripiprazole would be a good starting option. If she does not agree to an informal admission, she can be admitted on the basis of her parents' agreement. However, it is usually better practice to use the Mental Health Act as it affords the girl greater protection of her rights. Whether she is admitted or not will depend in part on her risk and also how the family is able to manage this and keep her safe. Electroconvulsive therapy (ECT) is rarely considered in people under the age of 18. She is likely to need some supportive therapy during the acute stage and as her psychosis settles. Cognitive behaviour therapy would also be of benefit. The family will also require support in how best to help the girl. On recovery, therapies and support that allow her to return to normal living are crucial and involvement of the early intervention psychosis team will ensure follow-up and relapse prevention.

Key Points

- Depression with features of psychosis carries greater risk of self-harm and suicide.
- Careful history taking is necessary with a need to be careful not just to take information given to you at face value – if what the patient says is incongruent with what you observe, keep gently probing.
- Where risk is high consider inpatient care.

CASE 83: SEEING THINGS THAT AREN'T THERE

History

A 17-year-old man attends the accident and emergency department with his girlfriend. He lives with his parents, who do not know he is here. She says that for the last 4 weeks he has been seeing things that scare him in the night. He often cannot describe them but they are large shapes that move and are accompanied with strong sensations of fear. She says he does not want to see any of his friends and is worried that they hate him and want to do him some harm. He explains that he has had panic attacks during the day and regularly experiences palpitations. He has increased his previous use of cannabis because this helps him feel more relaxed. His girlfriend says that one day she came in and watched him from the door. She found him sitting, rocking and picking at his skin and seemed to be in a world of his own. He admits that he has always used a range of substances including alcohol, cannabis, MDMA (Ecstasy), methylphenidate, temazepam, ketamine and dexamfetamine. His girlfriend says that he does not want his parents to know he has come.

Mental state examination

He is dishevelled and smells strongly, as if he has not washed for a while. He is furtive and does not sit still. His eye contact is fleeting. Occasionally he wrings his hands or rocks and then stops as if checking himself. He glances up regularly at his girlfriend and the cubicle curtain. He turns abruptly several times and looks at the oxygen port on the cubicle wall, and when you ask him what he is looking at he says: 'Can you hear that?' When you ask about this he says: 'mumbling and stuff'. You hear no noises of this nature. He looks frightened, and when asked says: 'I feel like death, awful'. He has some paranoid ideas about his friends wanting to harm him. His girlfriend interrupts to say that his two best friends care about him and want to help him. He looks at her intently but does not reply. He says he has no intention to harm anyone or himself. His insight into his problems is limited.

Physical examination shows a raised blood pressure of 145/95 mm Hg and a pulse of 100 beats per minute.

Questions

- What questions can you use to elicit auditory hallucinations?
- What is the differential diagnosis?
- What is the most likely diagnosis and the treatment?

ANSWER 83

A question to elicit auditory hallucinations is not 'Can you hear voices?' since this can mean many different things to different people. A clearer question is, 'Do you ever hear any noises or voices when there is no-one around or nothing to explain it?'

In the differential diagnosis it is important to exclude physical causes. These would include hyperthyroidism, delirium caused by infection, alcohol withdrawal or a space-occupying lesion.

Panic disorder would explain some of the symptoms but not all of them. A paranoid psychosis such as schizophrenia is possible, but the most likely diagnosis is drug-induced psychosis. Amphetamine-like drugs make more dopamine available at receptor sites and are thought to be responsible for either provoking a brief psychotic episode or precipitating psychosis in someone who has a predisposition to it.

The treatment includes a decision to stop using the drug that is leading to the problem. Motivational interviewing may help. A period of observation during this time is helpful. Ideally no medication would be used unless the young person was highly agitated or distressed in which case medication can be used symptomatically. Dopamine-blocking antipsychotic medication such as olanzapine, risperidone or quetiapine may be used if symptoms do not abate.

Treatment includes close monitoring and is likely to require admission to hospital or some intense home treatment. If the patient poses a risk to himself or others, use of the Mental Health Act and hospital admission should be considered. If the patient is on medication, side-effects should be monitored. The care plan should include consideration of the patient's family and his social needs. Support will be needed to help him regain his confidence and a relapse prevention plan will need to be drawn up once recovery is underway. This would include psychoeducational work and lifestyle changes.

He is 17 and so can consent in his own right if he has capacity. It will be important to assess this. You will need to involve the child mental health service (although he can also choose to see the adult services if he prefers). It is good practice to involve the family as they can help in the recovery, and it will be necessary to sensitively explore why he does not want to inform his parents. If they are likely to be supportive then gentle discussion with him and his girlfriend about involving the family should take place.

Key Points

- Drugs that make more dopamine available at receptor sites can provoke psychosis.
- Drug-induced psychosis can occur from a range of psychoactive substances that are both prescribed and illegally obtained.
- Mesolimbic and other dopaminergic pathways are thought to be affected.
- Delusions and auditory, visual and rarely tactile hallucinations may occur. Cognitive effects (including thought disorder) may occur.
- Relapse prevention work is essential.
- Dopamine-blocking medication should be used if abstinence from the offending medication does not lead to improvement.

CASE 84: SHE IS SO CLINGY. IT'S LIKE HAVING A SHADOW

History

A 7-year-old girl presents with a poor track record of school attendance. Her mother struggles to get her to school because the girl is constantly tearful. Her mother reports that her daughter has always been a somewhat anxious and sensitive child. When she was a toddler she used to get very upset if her mother was not constantly with her. It was so difficult that her mother gave up her job and became a nursery assistant to ensure the girl went to nursery. She had hoped things would improve as her daughter got older but in fact things are now worse than ever. Her daughter is reluctant to be looked after by anyone other than her mother, and cries constantly if her mother is not visible to her. She will not sleep in her own room and by the morning has often worked her way to her parents' room or bed. This is causing some marital tension as the father feels the girl is this way because her mother is too soft. Her mother states that there is nothing of note in the girl's early history except that when she was about 3 her mother had a few days in hospital. She wonders if the clinginess became worse when she returned home.

Mental state examination

The girl is reluctant to talk with you or join you in playing with the toys in your room. She sits almost on top of her mother clinging to her. The mere suggestion that she might be seen alone elicits floods of tears and she is almost inconsolable. When she is persuaded by her mother with a lot of coaxing to speak, she avoids eye contact with you and addresses her mother. She talks in a babyish voice. After continued encouragement she says a few words to you. There is still no eye contact and she remains in close physical contact with her mother.

Questions

- What is the likely diagnosis?
- How would you manage this?

ANSWER 84

The most likely diagnosis is separation anxiety disorder which is more common in girls and is most notable around the time of starting school. There is a need to exclude a general anxiety condition and any other anxieties as these often coexist. It is also worth considering if there have been any recent life events that might have exacerbated an already difficult situation. Children who have been traumatized or abused may be very clingy and anxious. Autism spectrum disorder may also need to be excluded because there are high levels of anxiety in some as they struggle to cope with social situations.

It is likely that there may be a strong family history of anxiety and/or mood disorders. Children with separation anxiety disorder are at greater risk of developing mood disorders and other anxiety disorders such as panic disorder, social phobia and/or agoraphobia in later life. Separation anxiety is developmentally normal from about 7–9 months of age and declines with time, but separation anxiety disorder goes on for longer and can interfere with social functioning. It can be understood from an attachment theory perspective.

The treatment of choice is systemic therapy or cognitive behaviour therapy (CBT) in a family context. The family and other adults will need education around the developmental needs of the child in terms of the development of resilience in the face of anxieties and how as parents to support this. The strategies parents sometimes use of protecting the child from the anxiety or repeated reassurance may reduce coping and reinforce rather than allay the anxiety. In shorter-term cases a straightforward behavioural management plan may be all that is required after careful explanations and support to the family. Useful techniques to use can be positive self-talk, coping strategy work and cognitive techniques to explore different ways of looking at the issue. Encouraging open communication and discussion of difficult situations with problem solving can empower many children. Relaxation techniques such as visualization can be particularly useful. It is also worth educating the family that such anxieties are more likely to return when there is increased stress. Being aware of this can help identify the problem earlier and enable the young person and family to use previously learnt interventions to prevent escalation. It is common for such problems when they have resolved to return in periods of transition.

Key Points

- Separation anxiety usually has a long history.
- There is often a strong history of anxiety in the family which may necessitate family therapy and/or family work.
- Coping and resilience need to be encouraged in an empowering way.

CASE 85: SOILING BEHIND SOFA

History

An 11-year-old boy is presented with soiling in different places throughout the house, for example, in the living room behind the sofa. He has been doing this for some years but the situation has recently worsened. He also wets at night and urinates in inappropriate places. He does not appear to be wet during the day.

The boy is currently in temporary foster care while his future care is planned. He was removed from his mother's care because there was some concern over whether she could meet his emotional needs after several episodes of emotional abuse and neglect. She herself has a moderate learning disability.

The mother had an uncomplicated pregnancy and delivery with the boy. However, when he was only a few days old his father left. His mother has always struggled to care for him. His development was initially delayed but he had a spell in care during which he made rapid gains. However, as his mother was said to have benefited from some parenting work he was returned to her care. His supervision by her has been very variable and he has often had to fend for himself. Attendance at school has been variable, but when at school he has shown a mistrust of adults and a tendency to be aggressive with his peers.

Mental state examination and physical examination

He is a wary boy who makes fleeting eye contact but then looks away. He does not willingly engage in questions related to the soiling but will answer questions about more general issues. He is somewhat small for his age.

Physical examination shows he has a small abdominal mass, and rectal examination and abdominal X-ray show that he is constipated.

Question

- How would you manage this situation?

ANSWER 85

Differential diagnosis would include constipation and anal fissure causing retention and leading to a vicious cycle of bowel loading and dysfunction. However, the deliberate soiling and the history suggest emotional and behavioural disturbance. Attachment problems are likely given the history of current neglect and history of abuse. It is possible that the extent of abuse is more than has been discovered. Rare physical causes like short-loop Hirschsprung disease, if considered, would require referral to a paediatrician. This would be sensible if constipation is ongoing. The smearing is not likely to be organic, but physical and psychological causes can coexist. In many respects the behaviour represents maladaptive coping strategies.

! Medical causes for faecal soiling

These include functional constipation and faecal retention, anorectal lesions that make defecation painful, neurological causes, bowel disease, endocrine or metabolic causes.

Encopresis (involuntary soiling) is more likely to occur in boys than girls. It tends to improve with age and is relatively uncommon after age 16. Most children with encopresis have learnt to control their bowels, but for various reasons lose this ability and develop secondary encopresis.

Management will usually begin with treatment of any constipation and reinstatement of an effective training strategy with support for the carers. Cognitive behaviour therapy (CBT) and contingency strategies are useful. However, any underlying psychiatric disorder will need to be treated or managed (such as counselling for past abuse) although this can be more difficult the older the child is. It is also important to be aware that encopresis may lead to scapegoating, anxiety and low self-esteem. Addressing these will also need to be part of the overall management strategy. The initial treatment can begin immediately and supporting treatments can be undertaken simultaneously. Child protection issues need to be reviewed, particularly as these behaviours may represent a 'flag' for emotional or family disturbance that needs to be addressed.

Key Points

- Faecal smearing should alert professionals that there may be child protection issues to consider.
- Treatment of the constipation will not be sufficient.

CASE 86: SHE WON'T SAY ANYTHING AT SCHOOL

History

A 10-year-old girl is brought to her general practitioner by her mother. Her mother says that she has always been shy, but her school reports that she has not spoken in class for several months. She comes from a close-knit family and she has grandparents as well as uncles, aunts and cousins living near by. Her mother reports that she chats happily with them all and with the nuclear family. She is the eldest of two girls and her sister is reported as having no problems. Her father is reported as being a shy, 'reserved' man who works for a gas production company.

At school she has one close friend who she plays with at playtime (including observed imaginative play) but no other real friends. In class, when the teacher asks her a question she remains silent and looks so uncomfortable that the teachers have taken to avoiding asking her questions. She will happily get on with her work and follows instructions. She does not have any significant learning difficulties that the school is aware of and gets 'average' marks in most subjects.

Her mother says that she has not had any illnesses or symptoms recently that she is concerned about. She has been sleeping and eating well. She takes a packed lunch to school and it is always finished.

Mental state examination

She comes into surgery with her mother but does not look at the doctor very much and remains silent, even when directly asked straightforward questions. She does not smile and her facial expression is neutral. She is smartly dressed, with neat, clean hair in a pony tail. She shows no signs of restlessness, agitation or slowness of movements. She is reported as being happy and chatty at home. Her mother reports no unusual or strange behaviour recently, and she is not distracted or responding to voices. She has no outward signs of illness.

Questions

- What possible causes are there?
- What further questions would you ask to exclude potential causes?
- How might she be treated?

ANSWER 86

The most likely cause is elective mutism (sometimes called selective mutism). This is where a child selectively withdraws speech from one setting in their life. It is not uncommon for this to be at school. However, it is important to exclude other causes of loss of speech including brain injury, epilepsy or encephalitis. These are unlikely given the history but you would ask about fits, faints, dizzy spells, headaches, vomiting, loss of power or sensation, fever and other intercurrent illnesses. Autism spectrum disorders should be considered since conversational reciprocity problems are common in those with Asperger syndrome. Further questions about social, imaginative and communicative skills will be important as will questions about the ability of the 10-year-old to empathize with others (e.g. when they are hurt, ill or upset). Depression and psychosis should be excluded as should obsessive-compulsive disorder, all of which can lead to withdrawal of speech. A post-traumatic reaction must also be excluded since the research has shown that children who have been abused can become mute in some or all settings. Getting to know the family, including a home visit, can give clues about this. If you have concerns then local children's social services keep registers of concerns raised about children by other professionals and this may give you further information. A referral to a child mental health professional (child psychiatrist or child psychologist) seems likely and they would be able to explore this problem further in individual or family work.

Many children, however, seem to develop this condition without any specific trauma, and it is likely that genetics and temperament play a part. A situational silence may occur over a period of time in the context, for example, of embarrassment. This can then become a habit that forms and is difficult to break.

! Criteria that establish diagnosis of elective mutism

- Absence of speech in a certain area of life (e.g. school) that goes on for at least one month.
- Interference with educational or social functioning.
- The problem is not as a result of anxiety about using a foreign language or about a speech impediment, and is not as a result of another mental illness such as psychosis, an autism spectrum disorder, depression or obsessive-compulsive disorder.

Treatment should be instituted as early as possible, as the longer the problem continues the more difficult it may be to achieve improvement. The main treatment is desensitization. This can involve the environment, the people or the communication type. For example, the environment in which a child speaks may be gradually extended. Similarly, if the child regularly talks to another person (e.g. a sibling) desensitization may introduce other people into that situation (e.g. a best friend initially and so on). Finally, the communication type may be changed to give the child a range of new communicative experiences (e.g. using texting, instant messaging on a computer, email etc.) Sometimes family work may help although this needs to be done with some skill, since over-focus on the symptom can reinforce it, and so many clinicians may focus on other goals such as establishing new friendships or developing confidence, rather than the mutism. A focus on developing confidence through achievement can also lead to benefits.

Key Points

- Exclude other potential causes.
- Treat early to prevent the problem becoming entrenched.

CASE 87: CHECKING

History

A 10-year-old boy is brought to the general practitioner (GP) by his father. His father describes that his son has developed facial grimacing and tics 6 weeks ago having not had them before this. At the same time he has started checking things in the house. For example, he checks the back door is locked repetitively in the evenings. He also repetitively touches radiators in every room over and over again. He becomes irritable if it is mentioned. It is taking him longer to get ready for school and at bedtime, apparently because he is following routines and repeating them. He is also more lethargic recently and needs more sleep. The boy himself cannot explain why he needs to do these things, and says that he cannot help the movements. His father says that he was well until 6 weeks ago and before this none of these behaviours were present. He says that he was very ill with a sore throat and fever 8 weeks ago and had a week off school. He has not had time off school for several years prior to this. His father wonders if the illness has unsettled his routine or whether there is something bothering him at school although the boy himself says that he has no worries about school. He has a number of friends. His father says that he himself used to have a blinking tic when he was about 8 or 9 and he grew out of it.

You do not carry out an examination, but note that the boy has facial tics regularly throughout the meeting that involve spasms of the neck and blinking, as well as some facial grimacing. He is slightly anxious to be seeing you, but no more than many boys you see.

Question

- What do you think is going on?

ANSWER 87

Transient tic disorder (regular tics that have been present for less than 12 months) is common in children and young people and will often burn itself out with time. It usually involves blinking or jerking of the head and the advice to family and teachers is not to focus too much attention on it and to reassure the child that it will go away of its own accord. Worry from parent or child drives negative or anxious interactions that at best do not help and at worst may make things worse. A family history of tics is common.

Definitions

- A *simple tic* is a sudden movement of discrete muscle groups that repeats itself at intervals. A phonic tic is the same involving sounds. Complex motor tics involve more muscle groups. The definitions of complex motor tics and stereotypies blur into each other.
- A *stereotypy* is a complex integrated set of movements such as body-rocking. It may be present more in certain emotional states such as excitement or anxiety, and occurs more often (although not exclusively) in people with learning disabilities and autism spectrum conditions.
- A *mannerism* is a functional movement carried out in an atypical or unusual way.
- A *compulsive movement* is an internal desire to do something, often initially resisted, and it may be repetitive, as the compulsive cycle repeats itself.

Obsessive-compulsive disorder should be considered. The infection at the outset of this boy's problems may be important, since this young person has no history of these problems. Consider PANDAS (paediatric autoimmune neuro-psychiatric disorders associated with *Streptococcus*). This is a rare autoimmune-mediated response to group A beta-haemolytic streptococcal infection that is associated with pharyngitis following acute onset of obsessions and compulsions and/or tics with relapsing and remitting symptoms including emotional lability, anxiety, ritualized behaviours, oppositional behaviours and sometimes movement problems such as overactivity or lethargy.

The presence of obsessive or compulsive phenomena may require child mental health service involvement. In the first instance some cognitive behavioural treatment would be appropriate with follow-up. If this is ineffective then a serotonin reuptake inhibitor should be considered. For severe PANDAS some clinicians have suggested use of immunoglobulins, or penicillin prophylaxis to prevent exacerbations during future streptococcal infections, but there have been no randomized controlled trials to test these treatments.

Key Points

- PANDAS is a rare association between streptococcal infection and an autoimmune response leading to obsessions, compulsions and tics.

CASE 88: NOT EATING, MOVING OR SPEAKING

History

You are called to see a 13-year-old girl who has been bed-bound for a week. Her parents are frantically worried because she has not been speaking or moving at all for the last 2 days. She has not eaten anything for 2 days although she will drink from a baby cup regularly. You have seen her previously in your general practice surgery and referred her to a paediatrician 2 months ago. She was admitted and investigated after a 6-month history of fatigue and occasional muscle and body aches. After 6 days in hospital she was discharged with a diagnosis of chronic fatigue syndrome (CFS), and referred to a CFS service that involved her seeing a paediatric community nurse together with a child clinical psychologist. The psychologist was unable to uncover any hidden stresses or symptoms of serious mental illness. She has seen the psychologist once and the community nurse has visited three times. They had set up a diary to record baseline activities, movements and sleep–wake cycles, but the situation continued to relentlessly deteriorate. Prior to this she has not complained of headaches or loss of speech, vision, power or sensations. The history taken shows that she was not low in mood. Six months ago she was attending secondary school and had a best friend (although not a wide group of friends). She has been teased at school in the past and she has been described by her parents as 'a bit on the perfectionistic side'. She is bright and near the top of the class in many subjects. Her father works for a government organization and spends a lot of time away from the family home, and her mother is a caring and kind woman known to the practice because she visits old people in the area as a befriender.

Mental state examination

She is lying very still in bed with her eyes closed. When you speak she grimaces and shouts, but forms no words. The curtains are drawn and her mother says that she cries out if the curtains are opened. She is not dehydrated. Her pulse is 68 beats per minute and her blood pressure is 105/62 mm Hg. She makes certain noises to communicate that she is thirsty and her mother can recognize these. They involve breaths and simple noises and grunts.

Physical examination

Her tone and reflexes are all normal. She has no neck stiffness. There are no unilateral signs. Pupils are reactive, equal and fundi are healthy. Her skin looks healthy and she is not dehydrated. It is not possible to weigh her.

Investigations

There are no new investigations available, but a very comprehensive screen on her previous admission showed normal full blood count, urea and electrolytes, liver function tests, thyroid function tests, blood sugar, calcium and phosphate. Serology for a range of rare viruses and other agents showed no apparent active infection.

Questions

- What do you think is going on?
- What do you need to do?

ANSWER 88

It is important to think broadly at this point. She may have a physical illness that has not yet been diagnosed. The tests suggest that this is not hypothyroidism, anaemia or a severe infective illness, although further investigations are warranted given the severity of the symptoms. Meningitis or encephalitis are possibilities, although again unlikely given the history, investigations and clinical course. She has no neck stiffness or history of headaches. Cancer is another rare cause and occasionally children with brain tumours or other rare cancers may present in unusual ways, although this has not been picked up in her recent admission. The severity of the symptomatology means that a magnetic resonance imaging (MRI) scan is advisable after assessment by a paediatrician or paediatric neurologist.

You should consider a severe depressive illness given the severity of withdrawal. There may be an unknown trauma or stressor in this girl's life that is not so far uncovered. Obtain a clearer picture of mood and coping at home and school. A psychotic illness while possible is exceptionally rare in a 13-year-old. Ask about symptoms such as hallucinations, delusions or thought passivity experiences that she might have described to parents. Occasionally children who are having panic attacks may withdraw into themselves, as can children who have experienced severe trauma such as witnessing murder or abuse or experiencing abuse, rape or severe bullying.

Pervasive refusal syndrome (described in a paper by Bryan Lask)* is a term that has come into wide usage to describe children who have no other physical or mental health illness but cannot move or speak, and often refuse to eat or drink. This is thought to be a type of conversion disorder. The theory is that it is not feigned illness but a bodily response to severe stress, although the mechanisms are not fully understood. Some have questioned the use of the term 'refusal' in this context given that it is not thought to be entirely volitional. There are however known to be psychological, physiological and behavioural aspects to the syndrome and a biopsychosocial model of understanding and treatment is thought to be the best approach.

In this girl the severity of symptoms and the rapid deterioration mean that admission under the paediatricians is the most sensible course of action. This allows for a multi-disciplinary assessment including paediatrics, nursing care, the child mental health team, physiotherapy, dietician and if available a paediatric neurologist. A full psychiatric assessment is advisable. The multi-disciplinary team can put together a coordinated rehabilitation plan. This would involve identifying domains, establishing a baseline and then planning the rehabilitative path.

! Domains to consider in a rehabilitative plan

- Nutrition
- Sleep–wake cycles
- Motor (posture, mobility, physiotherapy, activity)
- Cognitive stimulation (including sensory stimulation)
- Emotional/psychological factors
- Social interaction
- Family support

Key interventions will be to prevent the serious effects of profound immobility (e.g. contractures, pressure sores, intestinal and venous stasis, muscle wasting) and to establish the conditions for gradual and healthy recovery. Identifying psychological or systemic factors that help shape family-based supportive therapy will also help.

* Lask B. 2004. Pervasive refusal syndrome. *Advances in Psychiatric Treatment* 10, 153–159.

Key Points

- Pervasive refusal syndrome is a complex disorder. It is not an *International Classification of Diseases, Tenth Revision* (*ICD-10*) diagnosis and research continues into the mechanisms at play.
- Similar presentations may attract a range of diagnostic labels depending on the preference of local clinicians, and this can hamper a unified approach to treatment (e.g. encephalitis lethargica, severe CFS/ME, post-viral fatigue).
- Treatment is best planned by considering a multifactorial formulation including physical, psychological, systemic and social factors.

CASE 89: HE'S ONLY BEING FRIENDLY ISN'T HE?

History

A 6-year-old boy presents with his foster carer. The boy immediately approaches you and is over-familiar. He wants to sit on your knee and is keen to engage with you in rough and tumble type play. He has been with his foster carer for 6 weeks having been removed from his family because of ongoing child protection concerns. The foster carer reports that in some ways he is an easy child to manage as he seems to take things in his stride but his poor concentration and attention may make it difficult for him to learn basic skills.

Mental state examination

He is an overactive lad and struggles to sit still. He cannot focus on anything for more than a few minutes. He is physically inappropriate wanting to hug you and other staff and patients that he has only just met. He has no qualms about approaching strangers and talking to them. He is cheerful and joins in other people's activities without waiting for an invitation. He fidgets during his physical examination but is generally cooperative although needs to be coaxed to stay on task.

His speech is not easy to understand. He struggles with undressing and dressing himself.

Questions

- What is the differential diagnosis?
- How would the situation be managed?

ANSWER 89

The differential diagnosis is attention deficit hyperactivity disorder, attachment disorder, abuse and neglect, adjustment disorder, global learning disability or an autism spectrum disorder.

Broadly there are two types of attachment disorder identified. Disinhibited attachment disorder refers to children who do not develop a preferred attachment figure and who will go off with strangers. They classically have problems with emotional regulation. They are indiscriminate about who they form 'attachment' to and are inappropriately friendly with everyone, showing little wariness. Social interactions are also poorly modulated. Disinhibited attachment disorder is a diagnosis not often made, partly because of lack of clarity about it. Some of these children may be withdrawn with poor social skills and autism spectrum conditions (ASCs) may need to be excluded.

! Attachment disorders/attachment patterns

Attachment disorders are diagnostic categories (e.g. *International Classification of Diseases, Tenth Revision* [*ICD-10*] classification system) and not the same as attachment patterns. The latter are classifications of infant responses to the Ainsworth Strange Situation Test,* which categorizes attachments as secure, insecure (avoidant or ambivalent) and disorganized.

* Ainsworth M. 1978. *Patterns of Attachment: A Psychological Study of the Strange Situation*. Lawrence Erlbaum Associates, Mahwah, NJ.

Children with insecure attachment on testing, especially disorganized attachment, are at significant risk of later emotional and behavioural problems. Many children who do not form secure attachments may be institutionalized or have a lack of consistent care. However, attachment disorder may also be present when primary caregivers have suffered from adverse perinatal events. It is important that attachment disorder is not diagnosed without understanding the context. Children will show developmentally inappropriate social relationships and may also present as having anxious relationships with caregivers and/or disinhibited behaviour (behavioural problems, inattention, poor concentration, aggression) or asocial behaviour (lack of empathy or ability to see another perspective) in which attention deficit hyperactivity disorder or autism spectrum disorder may be mistakenly diagnosed. Learning disability may also need to be excluded as children who demonstrate friendliness to strangers may be doing so because they do not understand the contexts for different social relationships.

There will be no need to manage this acutely apart from raising the carer's awareness. The carer should discuss the situation with the child's social worker as they may benefit from further assessment. Treatment involves good ongoing parenting. Many specialist teams and looked-after children support teams use attachment models to advise parents about how to nurture and develop healthy attachments, and these are currently being researched. Given this child's lack of wariness he may be particularly vulnerable to abuse and clear advice about protection needs to be given to carers, school and social services.

Key Points

- Attachment disorder can occur in any family but is most likely where there has been poor child care or poor parental mental health.
- Children with attachment disorder often show behaviours that may be mistaken for attention deficit hyperactivity disorder.

CASE 90: TANTRUMS

History

A 7-year-old boy is taken to the general practitioner (GP) because he is having regular and severe temper tantrums. His mother explains that this has been going on for 3 months. It has gradually become worse to the point where he can be screaming for an hour every evening. It usually occurs when he has been asked to do something that he does not want to do, such as getting ready for bed. When asked if he has always been a difficult child, his mother explains that he used to be more biddable, although he has always had a strong character. His 5-year-old sister by contrast has always been placid. His father used to deal with difficult behaviour by clear and firm instructions. He had a close bond with his father, with whom he went fishing. His parents split up 4 ½ months ago. His father had an affair with a woman from work, and while he initially stayed in the house there were frequent and loud arguments, usually once the children had gone to bed. He then left to live with the other woman, a divorcee with one 15-year-old boy. He has had his son to stay on one occasion, but has refused to have him back because of severe tantrums. The 7-year-old boy has also been tearful, eating poorly and having some nightmares. There is no wetting, soiling or destruction of property, although he has been sent home from school on three occasions in the last 3 weeks, once because of a fight with another child and twice with tummy aches.

Questions

- What is the most likely cause of the boy's problems?
- What is the main intervention?

ANSWER 90

Tantrums are developmentally normal for children ages 2, 3 and 4. They usually occur in the context of the development of the child's empathy skills (known to psychologists as theory of mind), their place in the world and a struggle to understand that their needs cannot be prioritized at all times.

Tantrums that persist at older ages or are severe and prolonged in nature often lead to families requiring additional support. While this is not an illness as such, the World Health Organization (WHO) does categorize behaviour that is extreme in terms such as oppositional defiant disorder (ODD) for milder versions and conduct disorder (CD) for more severe problems that significantly impact on social, educational and family functioning. Severe and frequent tantrums can be part of both of these alongside other behaviours. The WHO lists 23 behaviours that it considers part of this spectrum of behaviour disorders. ODD describes a configuration of the milder of these behaviours including refusal to comply with requests, tantrums, blaming of others and other similar behaviours. CD listed behaviours include stealing, running away from home, use of a weapon and cruelty to animals.

However, tantrums can also be understood in terms of adjustment with disturbance of emotions and behaviour in the context of a significant stressor. The stressor in this circumstance is likely to be the disagreements and subsequent acrimonious separation of his parents. It is always important to ask about what is going on in a child's life when they are presented with behaviour problems.

Adjustment disorder usually occurs with significant impairment to social functioning and this is the case here. It usually begins within 3 months of the onset of the stressor and remits within 6 months of the stressor being removed. Many children do adjust to the separation of their parents but it takes time and patience.

The main intervention for the child is likely to be loving relationships with both parents. This means re-establishing a routine, giving the child a place in the lives of both parents and avoiding the 'triangulation' of the child where parents criticize each other, ask the child to spy or compete for the love of their child by abrogating themselves from their parental responsibilities or replacing emotional care with material rewards. Many parents realize this for themselves. Some parents are caught up in the acrimony and need support. This can come from parenting support services, family centres, relatives or child mental health service professionals. These would all focus on giving the individuals in the situation a voice and recognizing their distress while promoting coping.

Medication is not recommended in this type of situation. The parents should be encouraged to keep the acrimony and disputes to times when the children are at school, and sort things out as best they can. It may help to advise the parents to explain to the teacher what is going on. Good parenting practice such as clear boundaries, calmness, positive approaches (e.g. positive reinforcement of good behaviours and modelling of good behaviours) and consistency are key.

Key Points

- Adjustment disorder is common and should always be considered when there are sudden, severe or recent changes in a child's behaviour.
- It is important not to pathologize the child, but to recognize the difficult process the child is going through and try to establish supportive systems that promote coping.

CASE 91: HE WANTS TO BE A GIRL

History

The mother of an 8-year-old boy presents with concerns that her son keeps saying he wants to be a girl. She states that he has always preferred to participate in 'feminine' activities such as playing with dolls, being interested in dressing up and playing with make-up. He has been doing well academically but has started having more problems with peers because they tease him about his liking activities they see as 'sissy'. He much prefers playing with girls but sometimes bothers them because he insists he is one of them. He has quite a few effeminate mannerisms and he is often seen trying to copy female gaits and swinging his hips. The family had noticed aspects of these behaviours when he was younger but thought he would grow out of it.

His parents argue about whether anything needs to be done or not but his behaviour is increasingly impacting on many areas of his life. His father is also worried that they have caused him to become gay and feels that he has failed as a father. At times he accuses his wife of having babied him and caused the problem. They have two other children, a boy age 11 and a girl age 13. The boy is embarrassed by his brother and they rarely play together. His sister finds him interested in her clothes and make-up. She is mainly tolerant but can be irritated if he is too intrusive. She worries about the teasing and bullying her younger brother is subjected to.

Questions

- What is the likely diagnosis?
- How would you manage the situation?

ANSWER 91

Gender identity is a person's basic sense of self as male or female and is generally consistent with biological sex. Gender role identity is a person's self-designation as masculine or feminine. Gender role is a person's behaviour, attitudes and traits that are designated by a particular society in a particular context and time as being male or female.

Clarify the behaviours that cause concern and whether the child has any worries or concerns. It is important not to make the child feel guilty for how the child feels. The behaviours may present as early as toddler age when the child may show a preference for the opposite sex activities. This may also manifest by choice of toys, fantasy roles assumed in dressing up, choice of name and type of clothing. The child may also verbalize a desire to be of the opposite sex. Boys tend to be referred to services more often than girls.

A majority of the children who present with such behaviour will not be transgendered and surgery before the age of 18 is not an option in the United Kingdom. In fact, most such desires fade as children get older, hence the need not to make children feel that there is something wrong. Many children are simply exploring their identity and societal roles. Some, when followed up to early adulthood, will be homosexual or bisexual in orientation. For those where there is family distress or personal distress, support may be required and child mental health services are geared up to provide this. In some the behaviours or feelings are short lived, especially when they are related to a liking for specific toys (e.g. dolls) rather than any desire to be a different gender.

The approach to the boy discussed here would involve listening to the mother's concerns and providing her with the relevant information. She and the boy's father and other family members may also need advice about how they manage the boy's behaviours. Arguments and blame of others or self are common as the family struggles to understand the situation. Work with the parents may allow them to move away from blame. Some services recommend support groups. Avoid the pathologizing of the child. Long-term psychotherapy is usually not appropriate at this age since it implies a problem. Reassurance that it does not mean anything is best avoided.

Key Points

- Gender identity dysphoria is not common but it can prove distressing to the family and young person.
- It is important not to dismiss concerns but also important not to predict outcomes.

CASE 92: BLOOD IN THE URINE OF A HEALTHY GIRL

History

A 6-year-old girl is brought to see the general practitioner (GP) by a single mother, who also works in an old people's home as a care assistant. The child's mother is holding a jam jar containing deeply red urine. The mother explains that her daughter has been passing bright red urine for the last week. She says that she has been screaming in pain when on the toilet. She also describes high temperatures.

A check in the notes reveals that the mother has presented the child 44 times in the last year, and while many of the visits have been for colds and other minor ailments for which there has been evidence, there have been numerous occasions when the doctor has been unable to find anything wrong.

In the past she came to the surgery with her mother reporting fits when she was age 5. These were investigated extensively by the paediatricians. The mother reported them happening 5–10 times per day at home, but during a 3-day admission for investigation none were seen by any staff. Enquiry of school also revealed no evidence of fits. Her mother failed two appointments with the paediatrician and subsequently told the GP that she had not attended because the fits had stopped and had not re-occurred since.

Physical examination

The girl sits quietly on her mother's knee and makes no eye contact with the doctor. She is happy to be examined with her mother present. She has no abdominal or loin tenderness. Her temperature, pulse and blood pressure are normal and clinically she is not dehydrated, malnourished or anaemic.

Investigations

- The urine supplied in the jar has the maximum positives of blood, but no nitrites.
- No other investigations are to hand at this point.

Questions

- What possible diagnoses should you consider?
- What action should you take?

ANSWER 92

It is important not to jump to conclusions. She may have a urinary tract infection although it is puzzling that she has no fever or bladder or loin tenderness given the large amount of blood seen. Painless haematuria is usually of concern and always warrants further investigation. There may be a neoplastic lesion in the renal tract although the mother did describe pain on micturition, which is at odds with the examination. This will need referral to a paediatrician.

Another possibility is feigned symptomatology, in this case by the mother. This is another good reason for review by a paediatrician. The term Factitious Disorder by Proxy is used in *Diagnostic and Statistical Manual of Mental Disorders, 5th Edition* (*DSM-5*) and is sometimes called Munchausen by Proxy, although this term is only ever used cautiously in clinical practice since accusation without evidence may lead to litigation. It refers to a parent or carer presenting a child with symptoms that have been fabricated by the parent. This may be an attempt by the adult to elicit benefit or care for themselves or to harm the child, and is usually an example of both physical and emotional abuse (Table 92.1).

This is different from an anxious parent who exaggerates a child's symptom in order to raise the level of concern in the doctor for the benefit of the child. Factitious disorder by proxy is often associated with a personality disorder in the parent, where they are prioritizing their own needs over those of the child, and often putting the child at risk. This is a clear example of child abuse and would prompt a referral through the local child protection system.

Keep very good notes of consultations, signed and dated. Discuss with a paediatrician and/or the child protection team if your concerns are raised. Use the Common Assessment Framework. In confirmed cases the child needs protecting and the parent needs treatment.

Table 92.1 **Examples of child abuse**

	Physical abuse	Emotional abuse	Neglect	Sexual abuse
Deliberate	Assault (e.g. hitting, burning, scalding, biting, beating, throwing, stabbing) Reports of illness that subject the child to unnecessary medical treatment	Negative parenting or relentless criticism Damaging intimidation, threats or humiliation Harm to loved people, pets or objects	Deliberate starvation or privation	Child exploited by adult in any way for sexual gratification
Lack of prioritization or understanding of child's needs	Taking illicit drugs in pregnancy without thought for the child	Absent developmental nurturing Withholding child from school	Inadequate provision of food, drink, clothing or shelter	Exposure to inappropriate images or acts Invasion of privacy

Note: This is not an exhaustive list.

Key Points

- Make very good notes of history and presentation.
- Refer to a paediatrician alerting the paediatrician of your concerns.
- An admission may be warranted. While it may be what the parent wants, it affords a degree of protection for the child and allows more comprehensive assessment.
- If you have any evidence of abuse or have suspicion of abuse then follow your local child protection policy. One element of this would involve notifying your local child protection (safeguarding) team.
- Know your local child protection policy.

CASE 93: CAN I GET THE PILL?

History

You see a 13-year-old girl for a sprained ankle. As you are examining her, she asks if you can prescribe the contraceptive pill for her. She tells you she has been in a relationship with a 35-year-old man for nearly 2 months. The relationship has had some sexual activity already, but she now feels ready for full intercourse. Her 'boyfriend' is reluctant to use condoms, hence her request.

Her family background is that her parents are divorced with the father having left the family some 5 years ago. She lives with her mother and her mother's partner of 4 years. She also has a brother age 11 and a half sister age 2. Her 'boyfriend' is a friend of her mother's partner. She does not want her mother to know about the relationship as she feels her mother will be jealous of her. Her 'boyfriend' has asked her to keep the relationship secret so that it will be more special for them. She feels that as you are her doctor, you are also obliged to keep her information confidential.

Mental state examination

She has a swollen ankle but nil else of note. She looks slightly older than 13 and is wearing some make-up. Her dress is casual and appropriate for her age.

Questions

- What would be your concern with this case?
- How would you manage this situation?

ANSWER 93

This girl is clearly being sexually abused by the so-called boyfriend. The fact that he is 35 suggests that the relationship is not consensual and she has probably been 'groomed'. As well as being at risk of sexual abuse, there is a need to consider how she is being parented and whether she is being adequately protected.

It is important that you neither jump to conclusions nor dismiss what she is saying. You need to ensure that you have understood what she has disclosed but do not interrogate her or ask leading questions. Make good, clear contemporaneous records.

Every hospital and locality has an agreed multi-agency child protection policy, which will clearly outline how this situation should be managed. The principles of them all will be the same but they may differ in some of the details.

It is important to let the girl know that you are legally obliged to share your concern regarding her safety. This means breaking her confidentiality and telling the local child protection team. If she had said that she would share information with you based on a promise by you not to share the information, you would have to say that you cannot accept the condition. While it may prevent disclosure it also prevents you having to break your word which you would be legally obliged to do. It is important to explain to the girl the action you are taking and the reason for it. There is a need to identify whether there is an immediate risk to her or not and also how her disclosure is shared with her mother. As the maternal response may be difficult to predict it would be more appropriate to discuss the case with a senior colleague and with social services and take their advice.

Adults who abuse one child are likely to abuse others. You would not notify the alleged abuser in such circumstances (even if it were a parent). You would leave this to the experienced child protection team.

! Circumstances when confidentiality can or should be broken

- When there is a need to protect someone from themselves, for example, a child who is self-harming.
- When there is a need to protect a third party because of potential harm from the patient to the third party. (There may be a need to inform the third party and/or police.)
- When someone is being abused (physical, sexual or emotional) or there is a risk of this.
- When someone is abusing a child.
- When legally obliged to do so.
- At all times, the user is fully and honestly informed if any such action is considered.

Key Points

- As a doctor, you are legally obliged to comply with child protection processes.
- It is justifiable (and essential) that you break confidentiality if a child is at risk.
- Do not dismiss what is said but do not jump to conclusions either.
- Do not interrogate the child. The police are likely to want to collect evidence through a formal interview.

CASE 94: HE DOESN'T PLAY WITH OTHER CHILDREN

History

A 4-year-old boy is brought to the general practitioner (GP) by his mother. The nursery school has suggested she bring him and ask for an autism assessment. The mother is distressed. This is their first child and they have no nephews or nieces to compare him with. The nursery school says he sits on his own and bangs toys together. In the home corner he piles things up on top of each other but does not enter into the role-play that some of the other children enjoy. His mother describes that he has always preferred to play on his own if other children are around. He also has a fascination for things that spin such as fans and carwashes, and sometimes he will pick up pieces of string, paper or plastic and twirl them in his fingers, watching intently. When excited he jumps up and down on his toes or flaps his hands.

Examination

In the surgery he stands in front of the GP and types on the keyboard of the computer repetitively. He makes no eye contact with the GP throughout the 20 minutes he is there. After a while he looks out the window to the car park and says 'Mondeo' several times. He does not point or try to engage his parents or the GP in what he is looking at. The GP does not consider an examination is necessary.

Questions

- Is the mother right to consider autism?
- What underlying theories are thought to explain autism?
- What should you do next?

ANSWER 94

This boy has enough symptoms for you to seriously consider one of the ASCs, sometimes called autism spectrum disorders or pervasive developmental disorders.

The World Health Organization Research Diagnostic Criteria require there to be six from twelve areas of symptomatology. There also have to be two of the first four listed. These include the following:

Social reciprocity problems

- Problems with the use of eye contact, reduced use of gestures in communication, difficulty reading or using facial expressions in communication
- Poor development of social or peer relationships and limited peer play and interactions
- Poor ability to understand the emotions of others, understand social rules or social cues
- Poor shared enjoyment, excitement or pleasure or engagement in the interests of others

Imagination and language delay

- Delayed development of imaginative skills, role-play and abstract thinking
- Delayed development of language
- Unusual or repetitive use of language including a tendency to use repetition of words or phrases; poor pragmatics of language use
- Poor development of give and take in communicative interactions and poor conversational reciprocity

Repetitive and stereotyped patterns of behaviour

- Preoccupations with abnormal intensity or unusual intense interests
- Regular mannerisms or repetitive stereotyped movements or behaviours
- Liking for routine, sameness or compulsive behaviours
- Intense sensory interests or fears, or focus on repetitive non-functioning parts of objects; tendency to focus on details

Other diagnoses that could be considered would be a neurodegenerative disorder (which a paediatrician would exclude with a series of tests) or severe abuse (leading to a child entering into a very isolated internal world), but this boy has a range of symptoms that make autism by far the most likely.

Underlying theories include significant delay in theory of mind development (sometimes called mind blindness), problems with sensory integration (weak central coherence), executive functioning deficits, and differences in brain connectivity. Bad parenting does not cause autism. It is now well established that there is a strong genetic component and research is ongoing in this area.

A referral to the local diagnosing team or paediatrician is appropriate and most areas now have autism parent training programmes. While they do not cure autism they can lead to improved developmental pathways for children.

Key Points

- ASCs include developmental difficulties in social reciprocity skills, imagination, language and communication, alongside repetitive and stereotyped patterns of behaviour.
- Diagnostic interview schedules such as the Autism Diagnostic Interview (Revised) (ADI-R) and the Diagnostic Interview for Social and Communication Disorders (DISCO) are helpful, as is the play- and interaction-based Autism Diagnostic Observation Schedule (ADOS2).

CASE 95: TROUBLE IN THE CLASSROOM

A 10-year-old boy comes to the general practice (GP) surgery with his mother. His school has indicated that he has become increasingly disruptive in class. He has two older brothers, both of whom do well at school and have gentle and calm temperaments. Her husband left her over a year ago. The separation was amicable and despite regular contact with his father, she is worried that the boy is having some sort of delayed response to this.

The school's reports have remarked that although he was always quite an excitable and overactive child, he has been worse over the last 2 years. He has difficulty sitting still, runs round the classroom, finds it difficult to concentrate and is often in trouble for shouting out. He shouts bizarre things like 'warthog' and 'blue badger did it', often using a different voice to his own. To a lesser degree it has been occurring on and off for years but currently it is particularly problematic. The words he uses change over time. He may shout 'warthog' in repeated outbursts over several days and then use a different phrase such as 'Julie's knickers' for several days. Sometimes the phrases are rude and upsetting to other children and staff. He has shouted out names such as 'stupid donkey' and 'big fat witch face' but never serious swear words.

Staff noticed that he used to rapidly nod and jerk his head, pat his lips or make kissing noises when he was engaged in work. More recently his fidgeting involves him tapping his foot, kicking his leg out and reaching to grab the air. He has a very pronounced repeated blink involving much of his face.

For short periods he can control himself on request. The teachers have noticed that he finds this difficult and is usually more disruptive afterwards with episodes of explosive shouting and lots of rapid movements.

His mother says that his behaviour at home is similar but that until the school spoke with her she regarded it as 'just him'. She noted that it seemed to wax and wane according to his mood or stressors. He previously had lots of friends but over the past year he has not been invited to friends' houses so frequently.

Physical examination

Physical examination is unremarkable revealing a healthy 10-year-old of average height and weight. Neurological examination is normal. Blood pressure and heart rate are in normal range.

Mental state examination

The boy is clean and appropriately dressed. He makes little eye contact and is fidgety. He shouts 'rat face beardy man' repeatedly on two occasions. He had a further three outbursts with high-pitched squeaking noises and other sounds such as 'meep, meep, meep' and squealed 'pig, pig, pig'. His speech is otherwise normal in flow and content for his developmental age. It is not rapid nor is there any flight of ideas. When asked to sit down he obliges although sits on his hands and jerks his head backwards and forwards. He says he cannot help these movements. When asked what happens if he tries to stop them he says he can, but that he feels 'tight' and sometimes feels like he wants to 'explode' afterwards. There is no evidence of thought disorder, hallucinations or delusions.

Questions

- What is your differential diagnosis?
- What is the prognosis for this child's problems?
- What interventions could you offer?

ANSWER 95

History and examination have revealed a long course with motor and vocal tics and stereotypies, difficulties with concentration, attention, mood changes and obsessionality. Important differentials would include attention deficit hyperactivity disorder (ADHD), obsessive-compulsive disorder (OCD), depressive disorder or complex partial seizures. This is not conduct disorder because behaviours are different in quality from the aggressive, destructive and deceitful behaviours that characterize it. It would be important to consider an adjustment reaction given the breakup of his parents' marriage. Even if not the main cause this could be an aggravating factor to his other problems. This should be sensitively explored.

Clues to the diagnosis come from the nature of the movements and noises. They are not malicious and they trouble him. Simple tics are localized and brief, and produce jerking-type movements. Stereotyped movements (sometimes called complex tics) involve more muscle groups and last longer. They can be in the motor or phonic domain. This boy is exhibiting multiple simple (squeaks) and complex ('rat face beardy man') phonic tics and multiple simple (head nodding) and complex (grabbing movements) motor tics. Suppressibility (shown here) is a key feature of a tic and can help distinguish it from other movement disorders.

Classification of tic disorders covers two areas: idiopathic tic disorders and neurological disorders with tics as a symptom. The latter group includes neurodegenerative disorders such as Huntington disease or Wilson disease, metabolic disorders such as Lesch–Nyhan syndrome, homocystinuria and neuroacanthocytosis. Arrest or regression in cognitive abilities would be a worrying sign that a more sinister degenerative or structural brain lesion was implicated. Cognitive and neurological examination should be carried out including slit lamp examination and blood tests for thyroid function, copper studies and acanthocytes. Sinister features in addition to intellectual impairment would include late onset of symptoms, a progressive rather than waxing and waning course, fixed dystonias, specific dysmorphic features (e.g. indicating fragile X or Down syndrome) and other focal neurology.

Transient tic disorder lasts less than a year and chronic tic disorder involves chronic multiple tics, motor or phonic but not both. Hence, Tourette syndrome (TS) is the most likely diagnosis here. This is also known as combined vocal and multiple motor tic disorder. TS starts before the age of 18, usually between 6 and 8 years of age. Under-diagnosed in some cases, there is a spectrum with many milder presentations. Tourette's original formulation described the shouting or gesturing of obscenities (coprolalia and copropraxia), although this is not always present. This can cause considerable embarrassment and distress. The aetiology of TS remains unknown. Gene linkage studies suggest it is familial in some. Basal ganglia and autoimmune aetiologies are being researched.

The prognosis is variable, but in most is self-limiting. It can wax and wane. On average the most severe tics occur at between 12 and 14, improving in late adolescence. Most people with TS still have tics in adulthood although they are often not impaired by them. A few suffer a persistent and disabling course through adulthood.

Management of TS requires time, good communication and a holistic patient- and family-centred approach designed to maximize the child's function. Reassurance and information about the lack of intentionality on the child's part are important. Education of family and school can prevent secondary problems including blame, stigma and ostracization, and can minimize school disenfranchisement. Focus should be placed on improving or maintaining functionality and symptoms treated accordingly. Psychological treatments such as massed practice or habit reversal are used but may not be effective. Dopamine blockade (e.g. haloperidol and risperidone) reduces tic frequencies, but rebound increases occur on cessation and side-effects such as tardive dyskinesia after prolonged use mean that caution is necessary.

Key Points

- Tics can occur in the motor or phonic domain, are associated with a premonitory urge and are suppressible.
- TS is the name often used for multiple motor and vocal tics associated sometimes with problems of attention, concentration and obsessionality.
- TS is usually a self-limiting illness that requires a holistic management approach. Education and support of families are vital and often more effective than pharmacological interventions.

CASE 96: RESTLESSNESS

History

A 25-year-old man with moderate learning disability comes to the accident and emergency department. It is 10 PM. His parents are with him. He is agitated and restless. He is unable to sit in the waiting area. His father explains that he had been on olanzapine for a year after an episode of psychosis where he thought the radio was telling him what to do, and he was hearing the 'shopkeeper' next door talking to him and telling him that he was a thief and a 'bad man'. His symptoms had abated but he had put large amounts of weight on. His consultant psychiatrist had changed the medication to haloperidol. There had been no recurrence of the hallucinations or delusions, but he had become highly restless 3 days after starting them and this had become worse over the course of the week. This involves him finding it very difficult to sit still and feeling anxious much of the time. Prior to this he had been doing well in a supported working environment where he works in a small team, making cardboard boxes. He has not been aggressive or described any intent to harm himself or others.

Mental state examination

He is pacing up and down when you see him. He is also wringing his hands and has fleeting eye contact. He will sit down, and is calm for about 3 minutes with a parent gently holding a hand each, and during this time he denies hearing any noises or voices when nobody is around, and does not hear the 'shopkeeper' any more. He denies any pain and says he does not feel good, but does not describe any specific symptoms. After talking for a short time he again becomes restless. He wants to leave. He returns to pacing.

Question

- What are the possible causes of his restlessness?

ANSWER 96

The causes of restlessness are many and include intercurrent illness, sleep deprivation, exhaustion or anxiety. Depression can also cause agitation as can paranoia in psychosis. However, you have no evidence that his psychotic illness has recurred and there appears to be a temporal relation with starting a new medication.

The most likely cause is akathisia. This involves restless movements with a subjective inner sense of restlessness. Fidgeting, rocking or pacing may be seen. It occurs with antipsychotic medication and to a lesser extent antidepressant medication and also in parkinsonism. Different studies report rates between 10% and 45% in neuroleptic medication.

The best treatment is removal of the causative medication. In this man it is clear that he needs antipsychotics. The risk of akathisia is higher in higher dosage and so reduction in medication dose is a possibility, although in this situation it is worth returning to an atypical antipsychotic such as aripiprazole or quetiapine, where the risk of akathisia is lower. Some clinicians have used benzodiazepines or beta-blockers. Anticholinergic medication has been suggested but is not usually effective.

! Motor side effects of antipsychotic medication

- Akathisia
- Extrapyramidal side effects
  - Dystonic reactions
  - Parkinsonism
- Tardive dyskinesia – involuntary, repetitive movements of the lips, tongue and face
- Tremor

! Other complications of antipsychotic medication

- Weight gain
- Diabetes mellitus
- Pancreatitis
- Hyperprolactinaemia
- Impotence
- Tachycardia
- Hypotension
- Seizures or reduced seizure threshold
- Agranulocytosis (particularly with clozapine)
- Neuroleptic malignant syndrome
- Flattening of affect, depression or dysphoria

Other potential side effects of dopamine-blocking neuroleptics include dystonias, which are prolonged and unintentional muscular contractions of voluntary or involuntary muscles. Neuroleptic-induced parkinsonism is characterized by the triad of tremor, rigidity and bradykinesia. It can look like Parkinson disease, which is caused by nigro-striatal degeneration. Another major side effect of neuroleptics is neuroleptic malignant syndrome (see Case 41). This involves fever, severe muscular rigidity, altered consciousness and autonomic instability. Mortality is high if not detected and treated. Tardive dyskinesia involves involuntary choreoathetoid movements of the mouth, head, limbs and trunk. It is usually a side effect of long-term neuroleptic treatment and can be irreversible.

Key Points

- Akathisia is a common side effect of antipsychotic medication.
- It is easily misdiagnosed as anxiety or recurrence of mental illness, and in the past was labelled as 'hysteria'.

CASE 97: A MAN WITH DOWN SYNDROME IS NOT COPING

History

You are asked to see a 46-year-old man with mild to moderate learning disability and Down syndrome. He lived with his elderly mother until he moved into supported accommodation approximately 2 years ago. He shares his accommodation with another person who has a mild learning disability. They both attend supported work placements 5 days per week and have support workers who sleep over at the house each evening and support them at weekends. The support workers are employed by Mencap. When you meet him you note that he appears somewhat confused about his whereabouts. The person who brings him to your appointment says that they have only worked with him for a couple of weeks but have collected together concerns from a number of staff which include the following. He appears to be more lethargic and less motivated. He is having difficulty coping with his supported work activity helping in the local café. On several occasions he has fallen in the house, once when climbing out of the bath.

He has left the house on a couple of occasions and has been found wandering around the local shopping centre. Members of the public have expressed concern that on one occasion he was noted to walk straight out onto a zebra crossing without checking if there was any traffic nearby.

His sleep pattern is very erratic. He often wakes at night and insists on getting fully dressed. He is complaining of abdominal pain and on a couple of occasions has been incontinent of faeces. This is very unusual for him and has caused him significant distress.

Mental state examination

Your first observations regarding him are that he does find it a little difficult to orientate himself to the room and has some difficulty sitting down in his chair. His eye contact is poor and he appears particularly anxious. You note that his verbal communication is limited. He appears to understand what you say but generally answers with a 'yes' or 'I'm not sure'. At one point he gets very enthusiastic about a wrestling programme that he watches regularly during the week. When you try to talk about the issues the care staff have some concerns about, he denies any problems in each of the areas, simply saying that he wants to go home. You do not observe any active response to voices or other unusual phenomena.

Questions

- What could be the cause of some of his presenting problems?
- How would you proceed investigating these?
- Who could you involve to further ensure his safety and well-being?

ANSWER 97

People with Down syndrome have a higher incidence of physical problems including leukaemia, thyroid disorders notably hypothyroidism, cardiac problems, chest infections and cataracts. Hypothyroidism may be the cause of his lack of motivation and work problems. It could explain abdominal discomfort, constipation and overflow. People with Down syndrome frequently experience periods of depression, particularly in middle age, and therefore one should explore symptoms of depression. This patient will require a thorough physical examination to exclude any physical causes that can contribute to behavioural and psychological change (e.g. cataracts). In addition, questions should be directed at important environmental changes including loss of significant relatives, support staff or day activities. The question of verbal, physical or sexual abuse should always be considered and asked about in a sensitive yet thorough manner.

People with Down syndrome are highly susceptible to Alzheimer-type dementia. The amyloid precursor protein is situated on chromosome 21. As a result of the extra chromosome 21 there is a gradual buildup in amyloid plaques and associated neurofibrillary tangles in the brain. Studies have indicated that the prevalence of dementia in people with Down syndrome between 40 and 49 years is between 20% and 55%. All people over the age of 40 with Down syndrome are likely to have significant numbers of amyloid plaques in the brain. The early stages of dementia are often indistinguishable from a depressive illness. However, the functional changes described and the changes in behaviour here are highly suggestive of early Alzheimer disease.

Complete a modified Mini Mental State Examination. Orientation in time, person and place should be assessed as should concentration and visuo-spatial skills, although this can be difficult in someone with limited verbal communication.

Obtain a routine blood screen including full blood count, thyroid function tests, liver function tests, B_{12} and folate. Assess capacity to consent and likely compliance with the procedure. If capacity and compliance are questioned and there is no urgent requirement, it is sensible to delay the blood test and work with significant others to develop a strategy. This could include taking blood in a familiar environment with known people and the use of topical anaesthesia (e.g. Emla cream).

Road safety concerns highlight a possible deterioration in his ability to keep himself safe. An assessment of risk should be undertaken and an appropriate risk management plan devised.

Make contact with the local community learning disability team. A psychiatrist who works with the learning disability team would investigate deterioration in skills and cognitive functioning and assess for Alzheimer disease. Consider anti-dementia medication following further investigations such as chest X-ray and electrocardiogram plus further assessment by an occupational therapist to include motor processing skills. These would be useful for a baseline measure of functioning.

Community learning disability team

- *Community nurse*: assessment of cognitive function and any evidence of dementia; liaison with existing support staff, support and monitoring and care co-ordination
- *Speech and language therapist*: assessment of communication skills; advice about presentation of information (e.g. verbal, visual, etc.); advice about strategies in the home (e.g. picture signs on different room doors if there is disorientation)
- *Social services care manager*: assessment of support needs at work and at home
- *Provision of additional funding* if required
- *Occupational therapist*: assessment of road safety skills and safety in the home (e.g. bathroom and kitchen) with advice

Key point

- Alzheimer disease is more common in Down syndrome and occurs earlier in life.

CASE 98: LEARNING DIFFICULTIES, BEHAVIOUR PROBLEMS AND REPETITIVE BEHAVIOUR

History

The mother of a 19-year-old man comes to see you in general practice hoping to understand her son's behaviour. She discusses her son's overactivity and behaviour problems. When he was at school these problems were often discussed at parent evenings. He found it difficult to concentrate during lessons. She also describes that her son can be unpredictable. A male friend of her husband suggested that he looked 'different' and she found this distressing as she had never thought this before. He had learning difficulties at school and received extra help in the classroom. A teaching assistant had wondered if he had 'autistic traits' but an educational psychologist dismissed this at a school review meeting saying he could be imaginative and affectionate. She describes how he always struggled at school, not just with his learning but with his friendships. She says that other children avoided him perhaps because he had some unusual behaviours. These included laughing out loud, repeating phrases and some repetitive behaviour. He used to be very preoccupied with the film *Toy Story* and talked endlessly about Woody and Buzz Lightyear who are characters in the film. When talking, he often repeated sentences, sometimes half a sentence or even a syllable at the end of a word. He left school at 16 and went to work with his father on the farm. His father gives him straightforward tasks 'because of his learning difficulties'. These include delivering food to pigs and cows and hens every day. He is reliable with these tasks and happy, but his father recently had a mild heart attack and his mother is worried about whether he could hold down a job without their support.

Mental state examination

He has poor eye contact but will look at you and readily smiles at you. He seems comfortable in your room. He is quite active, and picks things up and puts them down without much awareness that this might not be acceptable. He does not speak much but when he does he asks you if you like Doctor Who and seems pleased when you say you do. There is no evidence of any psychotic phenomena, anxiety or depression.

Physical examination

On observation, the general practitioner (GP) noticed the 19-year-old's high forehead, large head and long face. He has large, prominent ears and on inspection, the ear cartilage is soft. He wears glasses to correct his myopia (short-sightedness). The notes say that he has 'mandibular prognathism' but this is mild. The notes have also recorded a funnel chest, or pectus excavatum. His mother described that he has flat feet and very flexible wrists. The GP noticed that the 19-year-old chewed his hands when seated.

Question

- What is the most likely diagnosis?

ANSWER 98

This man clearly has learning difficulties. His behaviours seem continuous with earlier life and as such do not represent a deterioration, which might signal a mental illness (e.g. schizophrenia) or a physical illness (e.g. a neurodegenerative disorder or systemic illness). A learning disability is not a mental illness. Learning disabilities do affect social, educational and occupational functioning. This family has made provision for their son's abilities and found a role for him in the family that is productive and provides him with self-esteem and a role, all of which enhance his quality of life.

The differential diagnosis may also include an autism spectrum disorder or obsessive-compulsive disorder. The history and examination in this man may make you consider the possibility of fragile X syndrome. This is a chromosomal disorder affecting the X chromosome. When cells are grown in a folate-deficient medium, the long arm of the X chromosome becomes 'fragile' because of an expansion of CGG base pair repeats.

Women are carriers who can be mildly affected and men have the syndrome, which results in a variable phenotype. People with fragile X syndrome can be shy and have learning disabilities. They may have autistic traits and sometimes a diagnosis of autism. They often have poor eye contact. While there is a characteristic appearance with long face and protruding ears, and sometimes large testicles, appearance can be variable.

There is no cure. This begs the question whether chromosome screening is helpful and this should be sensitively discussed with him and his family. If he were to have children then his sons would not have fragile X syndrome since they receive their X chromosome from their mother. All his daughters would be carriers however. This means that discussion with a geneticist can be helpful.

Given that this man is happy living with his family, raising anxieties about diagnosis at this juncture may not be that helpful, and your priority given his mother's concerns would be around ensuring a healthy and happy future for him. For this reason a carer assessment may be the most appropriate. If they are not already involved then referral to the local transition team should make sure that he and the family are receiving all the help in terms of planning for the future that they will need.

Key Points

- A learning disability is not a mental illness.
- Transition planning is essential for people with learning disabilities to make sure that they have good planning to maintain their rights under the Disability Discrimination Act.

CASE 99: MALAISE AND HIGH BLOOD PRESSURE

History

A 45-year-old man from a group home with moderate learning disability is brought to the accident and emergency department. He has a fever and has been reported as having had a fit by a young care worker. She explains that he lives in supported accommodation and she has been with him today. She has only worked there for a week. She phoned the ambulance after she saw him shaking uncontrollably on the floor. She has phoned her manager who is on the way to the department. She said that the four residents had been having a small party to celebrate one of their birthdays. This man is not used to having alcohol and he had been drinking wine. He was well before the party and was eating heartily until he said he felt unwell. He complained of feeling 'bad' and 'sick'. He was also holding his head before he had the fit and said his head hurt. When she gave him a hug she said that she could feel his heart pounding. She has not brought any files but says that she knows he has seen a psychiatrist regularly, and that she was told that until about 5 years ago he was on several different medications for a severe and prolonged depressive illness, but that he has been well so far as she knows for the last few years on medication. She does not give him his medication and is uncertain what it is. She does not think he has epilepsy. It was not in her handover notes. His mother has died and distant relatives only visit very occasionally. Recently she says he has been happy, doing his usual activities, and there have been no concerns about him that she knows of. When you talk to the man himself he is alert but does not answer any of your questions. He holds his head and cries out occasionally.

Physical examination

On examination you are able to look at the man's fundi and see no abnormalities and no papilloedema. His reflexes are equal although very slightly brisk bilaterally. His pulse is 100 beats per minute and his blood pressure is 140/98 mm Hg.

Questions

- What is the most likely diagnosis?
- What further information do you need?
- What is the treatment?

ANSWER 99

It is possible that this is a seizure in a man with learning disability. Given common pathways of neurological involvement a person with learning disability is more likely to have epilepsy than a person without (e.g. about 30% in classical autism). However given that he has no apparent history of epilepsy it would be unusual for this to start at age 45 unless he has some kind of neurodegenerative disorder, for which you have no evidence. It would be prudent therefore to consider alternative options.

Seizures may be a sign of an intracranial lesion, but you have found no focal neurological signs or papilloedema. Alcohol intoxication can drop seizure thresholds. Consider the 'Cheese Reaction'. The history suggests that he was well until he went to a party. Since then he has had headache, palpitations, high blood pressure and fitting, and the symptoms have come on since he has eaten (possibly cheese?) and drunk alcohol. The cheese reaction involves hypertensive crisis brought about by eating tyramine when on monoamine oxidase inhibitors. This causes release of adrenaline. There is a risk of stroke if not treated and the crisis puts a significant load on the heart leading to increased risk of arrhythmias. This man's blood pressure needs monitoring carefully and no active treatment is necessary while his diastolic blood pressure remains below 100 mm Hg. The treatment carries its own risks since dropping the blood pressure quickly can cause hypoperfusion that can particularly affect the kidney, brain and heart. This man should be admitted. Depending on the time when the cheese was ingested then oral captopril or clonidine may be considered. If blood pressure rises precipitously then intravenous sodium nitroprusside can be used but only under supervised conditions (e.g. in a coronary care unit).

Given that you do not know what medication this man is taking, you should also consider neuroleptic malignant syndrome (see Case 41). This involves pyrexia, fitting and autonomic instability. You might expect musculoskeletal stiffness from this and it is not present. This means it is urgent that you find out what this man's medication is, as this will greatly simplify the options. Make it a priority to find out. Ask the carer to contact someone who has access to accurate up-to-date records, or contact the duty care supervisor or general practitioner for the home. Other possibilities include a panic attack but this would not cause fitting, although high states of anxiety can provoke pseudo-seizures. However, there is no evidence for recent high levels of stress.

After this episode it would be prudent to see if an alternative medication would be as effective for this man.

! Food containing tyramine

- Things containing protein that have been aged include
  - Cheese that has aged
  - Matured meat
  - Processed food
  - Fermented soy products
- Dried fruit
- Avocado and aubergine (AA)
- Prunes, plums and pineapple (PPP)
- Figs, raisins, oranges and grapes (FROG)

Key Points

- People taking monoamine oxidase inhibitors can react badly to food containing tyramine (hypertensive crisis) or tryptophan (hyperserotinaemia).
- A good medication history can be crucial in helping you to plan treatment.

CASE 100: COMPULSIVE AND AGGRESSIVE BEHAVIOUR IN A MAN WITH DOWN SYNDROME

History

A 32-year-old man with Down syndrome has lived in a group home for the last 18 months after his mother became too ill to care for him, because of diabetes, obesity and cardiovascular disease. He has been settled there and enjoys a new job in a supermarket. In the last month he has developed a series of compulsive behaviours including an insistence in the kitchen that everything is in its rightful place. This was not too much of a problem initially since he helped with clearing up after meals and did this systematically without it negatively affecting him or the others in the home. Recently however he has wanted to clear things away before they have been used. He has become insistent that things remain in the same place and that people do not move them. He also becomes very angry when anybody else moves things. This has caused arguments in the house and fights of a minor nature have broken out on four occasions. One of these involved a flatmate throwing a plate of food at him. The staff have noted that he goes around touching radiators and mirrors before he leaves the house and appears to have a routine that he has to complete. He will sometimes go back and start at the beginning because he has not been happy with one part of it. A new person joined the home 2 months ago and he gets on well with him.

Mental state examination

When you visit him in the home he sits on the edge of the sofa very slightly rocking back and forwards. When you pick up a newspaper from the table and put it back again he 'tut's loudly and then moves it so that it is lined up with the side of the table. When you ask him if he is happy he says he is and tells you about television programmes and musical bands that he likes. You can elicit no evidence of psychosis. He is not responding to voices and he does not say anything of a delusional nature to you; neither has he done so to staff.

Questions

- What may be the problem?
- How would you treat the most likely cause of his difficulties?

ANSWER 100

People with learning disabilities often need extra support in life with employment, housing and daily living. Learning disabilities are not mental illnesses, but people with learning disabilities are more likely to have a mental illness. A learning disability is an intellectual delay, and is often associated with syndromes or other difficulties such as Down syndrome, which is caused by a trisomy on chromosome 21.

This man appears to have developed obsessive-compulsive disorder (OCD). This may present slightly differently in people with learning disabilities, in that affect may be more prominent than cognitions in the presentation. People with learning disabilities may be able to articulate less clearly what their thought processes are in the evolution of repetitive behaviours, but often describe a feeling of compulsion or a buildup of tension. Because of this and the learning disability, the use of cognitive behaviour therapy may be more difficult, especially if the concepts are not made explicitly clear and explained in easy to understand ways with plenty of visual prompts and accessible information. For this reason expertise is required to deliver therapy. It may be useful to refer the person to a speech and language therapist for a communication assessment.

Always bear in mind that people with Down syndrome may develop dementia or cardiovascular problems and these should be excluded as causes of any new presentations. It will be important to look at the other potential stressors that could be contributing to this man's difficulties. Is he being abused or has contact with his family declined? Has his role changed since a new person joined the house? Is work going OK or are there additional stresses? In the first instance it may be that some interventions geared to making sure that he feels safe and content in his daily life could settle his symptoms. If not, a selective serotonin reuptake inhibitor (SSRI) may be helpful. They are less sedating, less cardiotoxic and have fewer anticholinergic side effects than tricyclics; and since people with learning disabilities may be less able or likely to report side effects they are the treatment of choice as antidepressants as well as in OCD. It is important to assess his capacity to consent to medication and to have clear monitoring of side effects.

! Side effects of serotonin reuptake inhibitors

- Nausea, vomiting, abdominal pain, diarrhoea, constipation
- Loss of appetite and weight loss
- Rashes
- Sleep disturbance
- Headache, dizziness, nervousness, anxiety, drowsiness or hallucinations
- Tremor, sweating, dry mouth
- Mania
- A variety of other side effects (check the *British National Formulary*)

Anyone taking SSRIs for any significant length of time should be withdrawn from them slowly to prevent unpleasant withdrawal symptoms.

A clear plan of support for this man would involve discussion with the family and between professionals with agreed goals and strategies.

Key Points

- People with learning disabilities are more likely to develop mental illnesses.
- SSRIs are the pharmacological treatment of choice in depression or OCD with people who have learning disabilities.

INDEX

A

M

N

O

S

T

U

V

W

www.ingramcontent.com/pod-product-compliance
Lightning Source LLC
Chambersburg PA
CBHW081211220925
32965CB00007B/227
9781138373761